HEART SOUNDS AND MURMURS

HEART SOUNDS AND MURMURS

A Practical Guide

Barbara Erickson, R.N., M.S.N., C.C.R.N.
Assistant Professor of Nursing
Youngstown State University
Youngstown, Ohio

with 59 illustrations

The C. V. Mosby Company

St. Louis   Toronto   Washington, D.C.   1987

MOSBY

A TRADITION OF PUBLISHING EXCELLENCE

Executive Editor: David T. Culverwell
Editorial Project Manager: Lisa G. Cunninghis
Editing and Production: Editing, Design & Production, Inc.

Printed in the United States of America

The C. V. Mosby Company
11830 Westline Industrial Drive, St. Louis, Missouri 63146

Library of Congress Cataloging in Publication Data

Erickson, Barbara.
  Heart sounds and murmurs.

  Bibliography: p.
  Includes index.
  1. Heart—Sounds. 2. Heart—Diseases—Diagnosis.
3. Heart murmurs—Diagnosis. I. Title. [DNLM: 1. Heart
Auscultation—programmed instruction. WG 18 E68h]
RC683.5.A9E73 1987   616.1'2   87-28238
ISBN 0-8016-1643-3

PTC/PL/PL 9 8 7 6 5 4 3 2 1   01/A/054

Dedicated to
Leonard P. Caccamo, M.D., F.A.C.P., F.A.C.C.,
mentor, friend, and inspiration

PREFACE

This program is intended for the beginning auscultator who wishes to learn the basics of listening to and interpreting heart sounds. The more advanced auscultator may find this program helpful as a review of the basics.

The format used is one that has proven successful in teaching heart sounds over the past ten years. Basic information in the text is accompanied by an audio tape. By first reading the text and then listening to the tape, the learner should have the essential information necessary to understand and recognize the normal heart sounds and the most common abnormal heart sounds.

This book is intended to be an introduction and a guide to learning heart sounds. To become clinically proficient in heart-sound recognition, the learner must continually listen to as many hearts as possible. Although the reproduction of heart sounds on the tape may be very good, it cannot replace the experience of listening to actual heart sounds. Please remember that the sounds on the tape have been distinctly simulated to facilitate learning. Sounds from real hearts are similar but never as clear as those on the tape.

The tape was made with a heart sound simulator using studio recording equipment.

ACKNOWLEDGMENTS

I wish to thank Leonard W. Fagnano, audio visual supervisor at Youngstown State University, for the many hours of work he put into the production of the original master tapes.

I am grateful to Leonard P. Caccamo, M.D., F.A.C.P., F.A.C.C., for his assistance in validating the sounds placed on the tapes from the heart sound simulator and for his many valuable suggestions.

My thanks go also to Mary Ann Bodnark, design supervisor, and Denise Donnan, graphic artist, of the Youngstown State University Media Center for redrawing my original figures.

INSTRUCTIONS FOR USE

The learner is advised to

1. Read the basic information found in the text regarding the sound.
2. Listen to the sound on the accompanying audio tape. The tape should be listened to repeatedly until the learner is able to discern the sound being described. Before proceeding to the next section the learner must *understand* and *identify* each sound being described.
3. Listen to the tape with a stethoscope placed about 4 inches from the speaker. For best results, the tape should be played on a quality tape recorder. The better the sound transmission of the recorder, the better the learner will be able to hear subtle differences on the heart sound tape.
4. Listen to real hearts. Practice listening to heart sounds over and over in order to gain proficiency and expertise.
5. Test his or her own knowledge of the content of each chapter by
   a. Comparing behavioral objectives given at the beginning of each chapter with his or her own abilities after completing the chapter.
   b. Answering self-learning questions at the end of each chapter and checking answers against the answer key provided.
   c. Listening to the "unknowns" on the tape at the end of each chapter and checking answers against the answer key provided.

CONTENTS

CHAPTER I

INTRODUCTION   1

CHAPTER 2

THE FIRST HEART SOUND (S₁)   16

CHAPTER 3

THE SECOND HEART SOUND (S₂)   25

CHAPTER 4

THE FOURTH HEART SOUND (S₄)   31

CHAPTER 5

THE THIRD HEART SOUND (S₃)   37

CHAPTER 6

MURMURS—GENERAL INFORMATION   42

CHAPTER 7

SYSTOLIC MURMURS   48

CHAPTER 8

DIASTOLIC MURMURS   54

CHAPTER 9

SOUNDS AROUND S₁   60

CHAPTER 10

SOUNDS AROUND S₂   67

CHAPTER II

FRICTION RUBS—PERICARDIAL AND PLEURAL   74

REFERENCES   81

GLOSSARY   82

INDEX   89

CHAPTER 1
Introduction

LEARNING OBJECTIVES

After reading this chapter and answering the self-learning questions
at the end of the chapter, the learner will be able to do the
following:

1. Identify the requirements for adequate cardiac auscultation.
2. Differentiate between the use of the bell chest piece and diaphragm chest piece of a stethoscope.
3. Identify two basic mechanisms of cardiac sound production.
4. Identify the four basic characteristics of sounds.
5. Differentiate between sounds of high frequency and low
   frequency.
6. Identify three factors that enter into the transmission of sounds.
7. Choose the appropriate area on the chest for auscultation of a
   selected heart sound.
8. Differentiate between ventricular systole, ventricular diastole,
   and atrial systole.
9. Identify the relationship of cardiac sounds to the cardiac cycle.
10. Chart heart sounds using the one through six classification scale.

REQUIREMENTS FOR AUSCULTATION

Auscultation is one of the essential aspects of the cardiac examination. In order to perform adequate auscultation, one should do the following:

1. **Use a quiet, well-lit, warm room.**
   To facilitate hearing the heart sounds, ambient noise in the room should be eliminated as much as possible. This means that room doors should be closed, radios, TVs, etc., turned off, and conversations stopped. Unfortunately a quiet room may be one of the hardest elements to obtain. The room needs to be well-lit so that the inspection aspect of cardiac examination may be done. Many of the heart sounds can be seen and felt as well as heard. A warm room helps prevent the patient from shivering and causing extraneous sounds underneath the chest piece of the stethoscope.
2. **Have the patient properly disrobed.**
   The stethoscope should always be placed in direct contact with the chest wall. Most abnormal heart sounds cannot be heard through clothing because they are lower in frequency and softer than normal heart sounds. Also, listening through clothing will produce sound distortions caused by the stethoscope rubbing against the clothing.
3. **Examine the patient in three positions—supine, sitting, and left lateral recumbent** (see Fig. 1–1).
   Listening in various positions will bring out certain heart sounds, especially some abnormal ones. For instance, the third heart sound (S_3) may be brought out by having the patient turn to the left lateral recumbent position.
4. **Examine the patient from his or her right side.**
   Being on the patient's right side forces the examiner to reach across the chest to listen to the heart. This stretches out the tubing of the stethoscope and decreases the likelihood of extraneous sounds caused by the tubing hitting objects (chest wall, side rails, etc.).
5. **Use a stethoscope with a bell chest piece and diaphragm chest piece.**
   This is essential for complete cardiac auscultation.
   a. **Using the bell**
   When the bell is held *lightly* (leaving no after-imprint on the chest) it picks up *low-frequency* sounds.

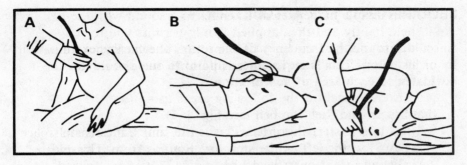

Fig. 1–1. Basic positions for cardiac auscultation. **A**, sitting; **B**, supine; **C**, left lateral recumbent. (Reproduced with permission from L. Caccamo and B. Erickson, *Cardiac Auscultation*, Youngstown, Ohio: St. Elizabeth Hospital Medical Center, 1975.)

Pressure on the bell causes the skin to be pulled tautly over the bottom of the bell and changes it to a diaphragm (see Fig. 1–2).

b. **Using the diaphragm**
When the diaphragm is applied *firmly* (leaving an after-imprint) it picks up *high-frequency* sounds.

c. **Differentiating frequencies**
The frequency of a sound is readily identified by noting with which chest piece of the stethoscope the sound is best heard. A sound best heard, or only heard, with the **bell held lightly is of low frequency**. A sound best heard with the **bell applied firmly, or with a diaphragm, is of high frequency.**

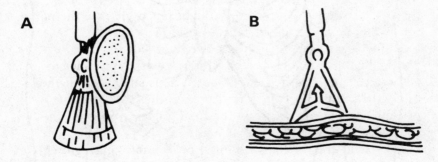

Fig. 1–2. A, *Lightly* applied to skin (no after-imprint is left) transmits *low*-frequency sounds. *B,* Firmly applied to skin (leaves an after-imprint) with skin pulled tautly over the bottom of the bell changes it into a diaphragm and transmits *high*-frequency sounds. (Modified with permission from L. Caccamo and B. Erickson, *Cardiac Auscultation*, Youngstown, Ohio: St. Elizabeth Hospital Medical Center, 1975.)

This simple maneuver of listening to a sound with the bell held lightly and then applied firmly permits you to determine the frequency of the sound to which you are listening. **This is an important point to remember.**

6. **Listen to each area of auscultation.**

Listen to each of the following areas using first the diaphragm and then the bell (see Fig. 1–3).

a. Left lateral sternal border: This is the fourth intercostal space (4 ICS) to the left of the sternum. Sounds from tricuspid valve and right heart heard best.

b. Apex: This is the fifth intercostal space (5 ICS) in midclavicular line. Sounds from mitral valve and left heart heard best.

c. Base right: This is the second intercostal space (2 ICS) to the right of the sternum. Sounds from aortic valve heard best.

d. Base left: This is the second intercostal space (2 ICS) to the left of the sternum. Sounds from pulmonic valve heard best.

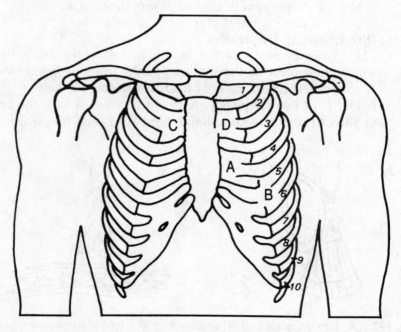

Fig. I–3. Sites for auscultation: **A**, *left lateral* sternal border (sounds from tricuspid valve and right side of heart heard best); **B**, *apex* (sounds from mitral valve and left side of heart heard best); **C**, *base right* (sounds from aortic valve heard best); **D**, *base left* (sounds from pulmonic valve heard best).

7. **Use a sequence for auscultation.**
   Each time you listen to a heart, begin at the same cardiac area. Listen to all four areas using the same order each time. This will help you establish a routine for yourself; you will "automatically" listen to all four areas each time you auscultate a heart.
8. **Use selective listening.**
   Listen to one thing at a time. When listening to the first heart sound (S_1), do not be concerned about the second heart sound (S_2). If listening to sounds in systole, do not be concerned about sounds in diastole. With experience you will be able to assess rapidly the total heart sounds.

CARDIAC CYCLE

The cardiac cycle consists of two periods: one of contraction (**systole**) and one of relaxation (**diastole**). During **systole**, the heart chambers eject blood, and during **diastole**, the heart chambers fill with blood. These events are readiy represented on pressure curves (see Fig. 1–4).

   Ventricular systole follows closure of the mitral and tricuspid valves. This systolic period is divided into two phases:

1. The first part of the systolic period has two subdivisions:
   a. This period begins with the first initial rise in ventricular pressure after the closure of the mitral and tricuspid valves. It is known also as the **isovolumic contraction phase**.
   b. This is followed by **rapid ventricular ejection**, which occurs when ventricular pressure exceeds the pressure in the aorta and the pulmonary artery. This forces the aortic and pulmonic valves open causing blood to be rapidly ejected from the ventricles.
2. During the latter part of ventricular systole, ventricular pressure falls and reduced ventricular ejection occurs. This period lasts until ventricular ejection stops and ventricular diastole begins.

   Ventricular diastole follows closure of the aortic and pulmonic valves. This diastolic period is divided into three phases:

1. The first third of the diastolic period has two subdivisions:
   a. Initially, in this period no blood enters the ventricles and

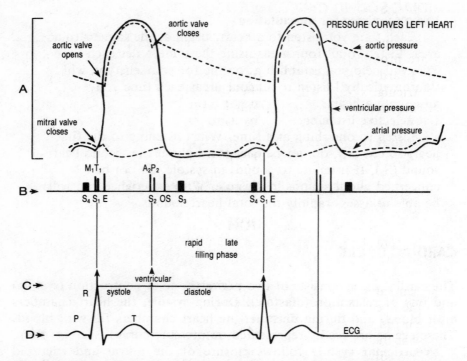

Fig. 1-4. Time relationships of various cardiac events. From the top down: **A**, left heart pressure curves—aortic, ventricular, and atrial; **B**, heart sounds—normal [S_1, S_2] and extra [S_4, ejection (E), opening snap (OS), and S_3]; **C**, cardiac cycle—ventricular systole and diastole; **D**, electrocardiogram (ECG).

    therefore, they do not increase in volume. This is known also as the **isovolumic relaxation phase**.

    b. When atrial pressure exceeds ventricular pressure, the mitral and tricuspid valves open and blood rapidly enters the ventricles. This is known also as the **rapid filling phase**.

2. During the middle third of the diastolic period, inflow into the ventricles is almost nothing. This is the period during which both atrium and ventricles are relaxed.

3. During the last third of the diastolic period, atrial contraction or "atrial kick" occurs and the remaining blood is squeezed from the atrium. This is also known as the **late filling phase**.

    Atrial systole occurs during the last third of ventricular diastole. Atrial systole may contribute 20% to 25% to ventricular filling. The contribution is less at faster heart rates (100 beats per minute or greater).

CARDIAC SOUND-CYCLE RELATIONSHIP

Cardiac sounds are named according to their sequence of occurrence and are produced at specific points in the cardiac cycle. The initial sound heard is the **first heart sound**, or S_1. It occurs at the beginning of ventricular systole when ventricular volume is maximal. The sound occurring at the end of ventricular systole is the **second heart sound**, or S_2. The period between S_1 and S_2 represents ventricular systole; the period following S_2 and the next S_1 represents ventricular diastole (see Fig. 1–4).

CARDIAC VALVE AREAS

Sounds from the heart valves (mitral, tricuspid, aortic, and pulmonic) are heard at specific areas on the chest:

1. Mitral valve sounds and other left heart sounds are heard best at the apex.
2. Tricuspid valve sounds and other right heart sounds are heard best at the LLSB.
3. Aortic valve sounds are heard best at base right.
4. Pulmonic valve sounds are heard best at base left.

The anatomic location of the valve and the auscultatory area (area heard best) are not synonymous (see Fig. 6–1).

   The amount of energy behind the heart sound's production is a contributory factor behind its auscultatory area. Since left heart sounds have more energy behind their productions, they are audible anywhere on the precordium. Right heart sounds, with less energy behind their productions, are usually heard best at only one area—the site to which they radiate.

CARDIAC SOUND PRODUCTION

Cardiac sound production results from at least two basic mechanisms:

1. The sudden acceleration or deceleration of blood, which is mainly influenced by:
   a. The opening and closing of heart valves
   b. Sudden tension of intracardiac structures (chordae tendinae, papillary muscles, or chamber walls).

2. Turbulent blood flow, produced when anatomically there is
   either
   a. Unilateral protrusion into the blood stream
   b. Circumferential narrowing
   c. Flow into a distal chamber of larger diameter than the
      proximal chamber
   d. Flow into a distal chamber of smaller diameter than the
      proximal chamber
   e. High flow rates
   f. Abnormal communications (ventricular septal defects, atrial
      septal defects, etc.)

These conditions can cause eddies in the vascular system and produce
vibrations that are audible (see Fig. 1–5).

Characteristics of Sound

Four basic characteristics of sound need to be considered: (1)
frequency; (2) intensity; (3) quality; and (4) duration.

1. **Frequency** is the number of wave cycles generated per second
   by a vibrating body. It is vibratory movement of an object
   in motion that initiates the sound wave cycles discerned by the
   stethoscope. Frequency determines **pitch,** a subjective
   sensation that indicates to the listener whether the tone is high
   or low on a musical scale.
   a. High frequency—the greater the number of wave cycles per
      second, the higher the frequency and pitch. High-
      frequency sounds are heard best when the diaphragm of the
      stethoscope is applied firmly so that an after-imprint is
      seen on the chest.
   b. Low frequency—the fewer the number of wave cycles per
      second, the lower the frequency and pitch. Low-
      frequency sounds are heard best when the bell of the
      stethoscope is held lightly so that no after-imprint is seen
      on the chest.
2. **Intensity** is related to the height of the sound wave produced
   by a vibrating object. Intensity determines the loudness of
   the perceived sound. High-amplitude waves are produced when
   an object vibrates with great energy; they are heard as loud
   sounds. Low-amplitude waves are produced when an object
   vibrates with low energy; they are heard as soft sounds.
3. **Quality** distinguishes two sounds with equal degrees of

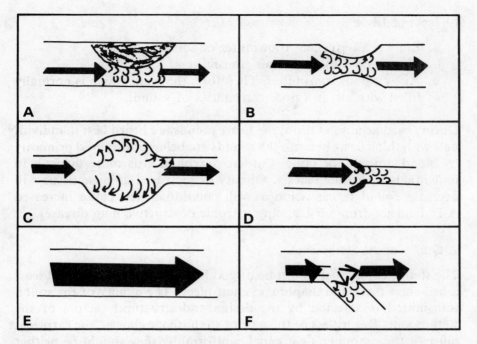

Fig. 1–5. Factors producing turbulence: **A**, unilateral protrusion into the stream; **B**, circumferential narrowing; **C**, distal chamber larger than proximal one; **D**, distal chamber smaller than proximal one; **E**, high flow rates; **F**, abnormal communications (i.e., VSD).

frequency and intensity, but that come from a different source (piano from violin or heart sounds from breath sounds).

4. **Duration** is the length of time the sound lasts. Heart sounds (S_1 and S_2) are of short duration. Cardiac murmurs or rubs are of long duration.

Each of the above four characteristics should be considered when listening to the heart.

SOUND TRANSMISSION

Three factors enter into how well a sound is transmitted from its source to the auscultator's ears; (1) the types of tissue through which it travels; (2) the quality of the stethoscope; and (3) the human ear.

1. Types of Tissue

   a. Bone is an excellent transmitter of sound.
   b. Blood and muscle are fair transmitters.
   c. Air is a poor transmitter. Therefore, the lung, which is normally filled with air, is a poor transmitter of sound.

During cardiac auscultation, the heart sounds are heard best in individuals with thin chests because the sounds are being transmitted primarily by blood, muscle, or bone. Cardiac auscultation is more difficult in individuals with thick chests. Obesity or increased adipose tissue will decrease sound transmission as will conditions that cause increased A-P diameter from air-trapping (chronic obstructive lung disease).

2. Quality of the Stethoscope

The stethoscope chosen must be of good quality and must have at least a bell chest piece and diaphragm chest piece. The quality of the sound transmitted is affected by the design and structural factors of the stethoscope. Regardless of the type of stethoscope chosen, the earpieces must fit the examiner's ear canal comfortably; they should be neither too tight nor too loose. The tubing of the stethoscope should be as short as possible for the clinical situation in which it is used routinely.

3. The Human Ear

Individuals differ in their ability to hear. The normal human ear is capable of perceiving sounds with a frequency of 1,000 to 5,000 cps and a duration of as little as 0.02 seconds. Because of the peculiarities of the human ear, high-frequency sounds may seem louder than low-frequency sounds of equal intensity. Also, very loud sounds may deafen momentarily. Therefore, the auscultator may have trouble hearing a soft sound that immediately follows a loud sound.

   High-frequency perception decreases with age, but this should not interfere with cardiac auscultation because heart sounds are in the lower-frequency range of what the ear is capable of hearing. This means the ability to hear heart sounds should improve with age.

CLASSIFICATION OF SOUNDS AND MURMURS

Sounds and murmurs may be classified on a one through six scale as follows:

1. Not audible during the first few seconds of auscultation; heard after listener tunes in
2. Heard immediately but faint
3. Loud but without a thrust or thrill
4. Loud with a thrust or thrill
5. Loud with a thrust or thrill and audible with the chest piece tilted on the chest
6. Loud with a thrust or thrill and audible with the chest piece just off the chest wall

"Thrust" is an *intermittent* palpable (sometimes even visible) sensation at the site being auscultated. This is the sensation felt when palpating the point of maximal impulse at the apex of the heart. "Thrill" is a *continuous* palpable sensation comparable to the vibration felt when a car purrs.

To chart a sound or murmur, a fraction is used (3/6 or III/VI). The numerator of the fraction indicates where the sound being described fits into the classification system. The denominator indicates the total number of parts in the classification. Therefore, a sound described as a 3/6 would be one that is loud but without a trust or thrill (as indicated by the numerator "3"). It is being described in a classification system with six parts (as indicated by the denominator "6").

CHARTING HEART SOUNDS

When charting heart sounds, a description of what is heard at each of the four basic auscultatory sites is given. Included in the description are the sound characteristics of frequency, intensity, quality, and duration. In addition the charting should include:

1. Area of auscultation—LLSB, apex, base right, base left
2. Heart rate
3. Patient's position—supine, sitting, left lateral recumbent, etc.
4. Description of S_1 and S_2
5. Presence of other sounds—splits, ejection sounds, clicks, S_3, S_4
6. Presence of murmurs—noting the following:
   a. Location of valve area where murmur is heard best
   b. Loudness (intensity) by using a one through six classification
   c. Frequency (pitch)—low, medium, or high
   d. Quality—blowing, harsh, rough, or rumble
   e. Timing—systolic or diastolic

Name _____ Date _____

AUSCULTOGRAM

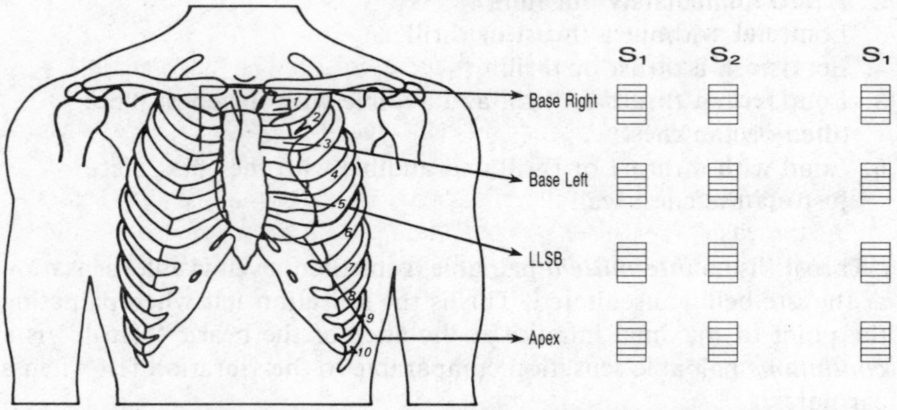

Indicate the loudness of the S_1 and S_2 at each of the auscultatory sites by drawing vertical lines to the appropriate height in the blank blocks using the one through six scale:

[Each block represents one classification in the grading system.
"1" being the bottom block and "6" being the top block.]

1. Not audible during the first few seconds of auscultation.
2. Heard immediately but faint.
3. Loud but without a *Thrust or Thrill.
4. Loud but with a Thrust or Thrill.
5. Loud with a Thrust or Thrill and audible with the chest piece tilted on the chest.
6. Loud with a Thrust or Thrill and audible with chest piece just off the chest wall.

* "Thrill" is a <u>continuous</u> palpable sensation comparable to the vibration felt when cat purrs.

Draw in extra sound [i.e. S_3, S_4, Ejection (E), or clicks (C)] as indicated.

Draw murmurs in the appropriate cycle.

Use the following sine waves to indicate the frequency/quality:

High Frequency = ⱮⱮⱮⱮⱮⱮⱮ
(Blowing)

Low Frequency = ⌁⌁⌁⌁⌁⌁
(Rumbling)

Mixture = ⱮⱮⱮⱮⱮ

Use the one through six scale to indicate loudness of murmur by drawing sine wave to height comparable to the loudness of the murmur.

Fig. 1-6. An auscultogram, a graphic method of recording heart sounds and murmurs.

f. Finer timing—early, mid, or late
g. Radiation—other area(s) where murmur is heard
h. Increase or decrease of murmur with respiration, position, special maneuvers, or drugs
7. The type of stethoscope chest piece used—bell or diaphragm
8. The effect of respiration or other maneuvers—inspiration, expiration, standing, squatting, valsalva, etc.

A graphic method of charting heart sounds (the auscultogram) is one of the easiest methods to use. The auscultogram provides an easy means of drawing what is heard during cardiac auscultation. The auscultogram includes the following:

1. A drawing of the chest with the four basic auscultatory sites marked.
2. Blank blocks drawn one on top of the other six blocks high. (Each block represents one classification in the grading system, one being the bottom block and six being the top block).
3. S_1 and S_2 represented by vertical lines drawn in the blank blocks to indicate the intensity of the sounds.
4. S_3, S_4, splits, clicks, and ejection sounds indicated if they are heard.
5. Murmurs represented by sine waves:
   a. Widely spaced for low-frequency sounds
   b. Close picket fence lines for high-frequency sounds
   The loudness is represented by the height of the wave on a one through six scale (see Fig. 1–6).

SELF-LEARNING QUESTIONS

Select the letter of the correct response or provide requested information. Compare your answers with the answer key at the end of the chapter. Reread chapter as needed to achieve mastery of content.

1. Name five of the eight requirements for adequate cardiac auscultation.
   a.
   b.
   c.
   d.
   e.

2. Cardiac sounds and murmurs of low frequency can be heard best by using
   a. a diaphragm chest piece
   b. a monaural stethoscope
   c. a bell chest piece
   d. either a bell or chest piece or a diaphragm chest piece

3. The two basic mechanisms of cardiac sound production are
   a.
   b.

4. The number of wave cycles generated per second by a vibrating body is a description of the sound characteristic of
   a. quality
   b. intensity
   c. frequency
   d. duration

5. The best type of tissue for transmitting sound is
   a. blood
   b. fat
   c. air
   d. bone

6. The frequency perception that is decreased with aging is
   a. low
   b. medium
   c. high
   d. none

7. At which area of the chest would mitral or left heart sounds be heard best?
   a. LLSB
   b. apex
   c. base right
   d. base left

8. The rapid filling phase, when the mitral and tricuspid valves open and blood rapidly enters the ventricles is a part of
   a. atrial systole
   b. atrial diastole
   c. ventricular systole
   d. ventricular diastole

9. The cardiac sound that occurs at the beginning of ventricular systole when ventricular volume is maximal is called the
   a. first heart sound (S_1)
   b. second heart sound (S_2)
   c. third heart sound (S_3)
   d. fourth heart sound (S_4)

10. Indicate the graphic representation of a cardiac sound that is loud without a thrill by drawing lines at the appropriate height in the following box:

ANSWERS FOR SELF-LEARNING QUESTIONS

1. Any five of the following eight responses:
   —Use a quiet well-lit, warm room.
   —Have the patient properly disrobed.
   —Examine the patient in three positions—supine, sitting, and left lateral recumbent.
   —Examine the patient from his or her right side.
   —Use a stethoscope with a bell chest piece and diaphragm chest piece.
   —Listen to the four basic areas of auscultation.
   —Use a sequence for auscultation.
   —Use selective listening.

2. c

3. —Sudden acceleration or deceleration of blood
   —Turbulent blood flow

4. c

5. d

6. c

7. b

8. d

9. a

10.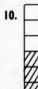

CHAPTER 2
The First Heart Sound (S₁)

LEARNING OBJECTIVES

After reading this chapter, listening to the accompanying tape, answering the self-learning questions at the end of the chapter, and listening to the "unknowns" on the tape, the learner will be able to do the following:

1. Identify the classical theory behind the production of S_1.
2. Differentiate between a single S_1 and a normal split S_1 (M_1T_1).
3. Recognize a normal S_1 at the various auscultatory sites.
4. Identify the physiological factors that affect the intensity of S_1.
5. Identify methods of differentiating S_1 from the second heart sound (S_2).

COMPONENTS OF S_1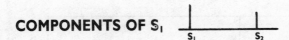

The classical and generally accepted theory for the production of S_1 is that S_1 is associated with the closure of both the mitral (M_1) valve and the tricuspid (T_1) valve. This classical theory is one of the easiest to correlate with the heart sounds heard at the bedside and, therefore, will be accepted for this text. Since S_1 is due to the closure of two separate valves, both valves must be considered when listening to it.

M_1 is the first audible component of S_1. This component normally occurs before T_1. (Left-sided mechanical events occur before right-sided mechanical events.) M_1 occurs just after the mitral valve closes. This occurs about 0.02 to 0.03 second after left ventricular pressure equals left atrial pressure. M_1 is of slightly higher intensity and frequency than T_1 and is discernible at all the auscultatory sites, but is heard best at the apex. Since it is a high-frequency sound, it is heard best with the diaphragm pressed firmly.

T_1 is the second component of S_1. It normally follows M_1 just after the tricuspid valve closes. Since there is less energy behind the production of this sound, it may be heard only at the left lateral sternal border (LLSB) the area to which T_1 radiates or is heard best. Since it is a high-frequency sound it is heard best with the diaphragm applied firmly.

SPLIT S_1

When both components that make up S_1 (M_1 and T_1) are separately distinguishable, it is known as a **split**. In a normal split S_1 the components making the sound are 0.02 second apart (see Fig. 2–1).

The separation between heart sounds must be at least 0.02 second or greater for the human ear to hear two definite sounds. Since the normal distance between M_1 and T_1 is *only* 0.02 second, a normally split S_1 may be difficult to hear. The ear may perceive it as "slurred" or "fuzzy" and not two separate sounds.

Listen now to an S_1 that is split at various distances. The initial split will be 0.08 second—the ear will hear two definite sounds. Gradually the split decreases—0.06 second; then 0.04 second; then 0.02 second (the duration of the normal split S_1). Practice listening until you perceive the difference between a single S_1 (only one component audible) and a split S_1 (both components audible).

In a normal heart, the split S_1 may be audible only when listening over the area to which the softer tricuspid component radiates—the left lateral sternal border. Although a split S_1 is common in children, it is

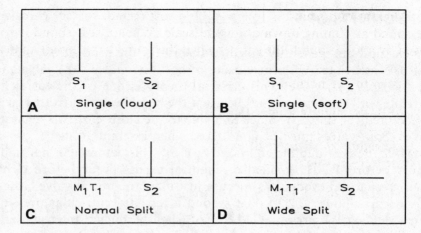

Fig. 2–1. Splitting of the first heart sound (S_1): **A**, single first sound (S_1) louder than the second (S_2); **B**, single S_1 softer than S_2; **C**, normal split first sound ($M_1 T_1$) 0.02 second; **D**, wide split first sound ($M_1 T_1$) 0.04 second. (Reproduced with permission from L. Caccamo and B. Erickson, *Cardiac Auscultation*, Youngstown, Ohio: St. Elizabeth Hospital Medical Center, 1975.)

heard only in about half of normal adults. To be considered a normal split S_1, M_1 and T_1 must be of high frequency and heard close together—0.02 second apart. The split is not affected markedly by respiration. When audible, it is heard consistently.

Listen now to S_1 at the various sites:

1. LLSB—split or single S_1 heard
2. Apex—single S_1 heard
3. Base right—single S_1 heard
4. Base left—single S_1 heard

INTENSITY OF S_1:

The **intensity** or loudness of S_1 also changes depending on the site auscultated. S_1 is always slightly louder than S_2 at either the LLSB or the apex. (The M_1 component of S_1 is heard best at the apex; the T_1 component of the S_1 is heard best at the LLSB.) S_1 is softer than the second sound (S_2) at either base left or base right. (The A_1 component of the S_2 is heard best at base right; the P_1 component of the S_2 is heard best at base left.)

When a loud sound is followed by a soft sound, the ear perceives the sound as coming **down** a musical scale. When a soft sound is followed by a loud sound, the ear perceives the sound as going **up** a musical scale.

Listen to the normal S_1 at the various sites:

1. LLSB—S_1 slightly louder than S_2
2. Apex—S_1 slightly louder than S_2
3. Base right—S_1 slightly softer than S_2
4. Base left—S_1 slightly softer than S_2.

When listening to a normal S_1 the following occurs at each specified site:

1. LLSB—Single S_1 or Split S_1, S_1 louder than S_2
2. Apex—Single S_1; S_1 louder than S_2
3. Base right—Single S_1; S_1 softer than S_2
4. Base left—Single S_1 softer than S_2.

The intensity of S_1 may be affected by the following physiological factors as well:

1. **The anatomy of the chest.** Sounds are easier to hear, and therefore, louder in patient's with thin chests. Sounds are harder to hear, and therefore, softer in patient's with thick chests.
2. **The vigor of ventricular contraction.** Sounds are louder when there is more energy behind their production, as occurs with tachycardia. Sounds are softer when there is less energy behind their production, as occurs with heart muscle damage (myocardial infarction.)
3. **Valve position at the onset of ventricular contraction.** If the valve leaflets are wide open when they are forced closed, as occurs with a short P-R interval, the resulting sound is loud. If the valve leaflets are almost shut when they are forced closed, as occurs with a long P-R interval, the resulting sound is soft.
4. **Pathological alteration of the valve structure** (stiffness of the valve). If the valve orifice is closed and fixed, a loud sound may be heard. If the valve orifice is open and fixed, a soft sound may be heard.

For a synopsis of the physiological factors that affect the intensity of S_1 and the resultant type of sound, see Table 2–1.

Table 2–1. Physiological factors that vary first heart sound (S1) intensity

Physiological Factors	Loud S₁	Soft S₁	Variable S₁
1. Anatomy of chest	Thin chest	Emphysema (barrel chest) Obesity Pericardial effusion Edema of chest wall	
2. Vigor of ventricular contraction	Tachycardia: exercise emotion hyperthyroid fever Systemic hypertension	Extensive muscle damage (i.e., myocardial infarction)	
3. Valve position at onset of ventricular contraction when valve mobile	Short PR (except WPW) when valve wide open with wide arc of closure ASD when tricuspid wide open due to volume load	Long PR when valve almost closed with narrow arc of closure	Mobitz I (regular sequential variability of sound.) Atrial fibrillation CHB A—V dissociation (irregular variability of sound)
4. Pathological alteration of the valve structure (STIFF)	Mitral stenosis* which keeps orifice closed and fixed	Mitral regurgitation which keeps valve open and fixed	

*When the first sound is *loud* and the heart rate normal, then *think mitral stenosis.*

(Reproduced with permission from L. Caccamo and B. Erickson, *Cardiac Auscultation,* Youngstown, Ohio: St. Elizabeth Hospital Medical Center, 1975.)

DIFFERENTIATING S₁ FROM S₂

When listening to the normal heart sounds, S_1 and S_2, it is important to be able to know which sound is the first and which is the second. The following suggestions will help in making this differentiation.

At a heart rate of 80 beats per minute or less, S_1 follows the longer pause. (The time between S_1 and S_2 [systole] is shorter than the time between S_2 and the next S_1 [diastole].) At a heart rate above 80 beats per minute, the diastolic period shortens, becoming equal to systole, and other methods are needed to determine which sound is first.

In a normal heart, S_2 is always loudest at the base. Therefore, listen at the base and determine which of the sounds is the loudest—this is S_2. Then gradually move the stethoscope from the base to the LLSB keeping in mind which sound is S_1.

Another method of differentiating S_1 from S_2, especially with a rapid heart rate, is to watch your stethoscope while auscultating. The stethoscope may move outward when placed at the point of maximal impulse and the sound heard simultaneously with this outward thrust is S_1.

S_1 can also be timed by simultaneously feeling the carotid pulse while listening to the heart. The sound heard when the carotid is felt is S_1. (Peripheral pulses **cannot** be used for timing cardiac sounds because too great a time lag occurs between ventricular systole and the palpated peripheral pulse.)

A synopsis of the methods of differentiating S_1 from S_2 is depicted in the algorithm of Fig. 2–2.

A big disadvantage of listening to heart sounds from a tape or sound simulator is that the physiological factor (carotid pulse) that aids in sound differentiation is absent. Therefore, it may be more difficult to discern S_1 from S_2. To make it easier for the learner to identify S_1 the rate of the sounds simulated will be 60 beats per minute unless otherwise indicated.

CLINICAL CORRELATION

After gaining confidence in your ability to identify S_1, hone your ability by listening to as many real hearts as possible. Listen to thin-chested patients and obese patients, and adults and children, if possible. Note the similarities and differences. Attempt to distinguish a single S_1 from a split S_1. Note the difference in intensity depending on the site auscultated. Can you differentiate S_1 from S_2 using the physiological factor

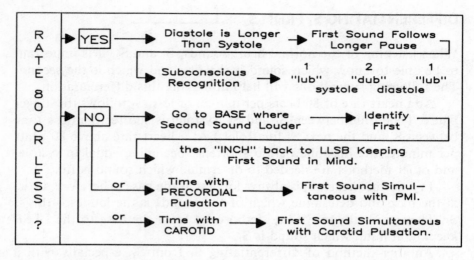

Fig. 2–2. Algorithm for differentiating the first heart sound (S₁) from the second heart sound (S₂). (Reproduced with permission from L. Caccamo and B. Erickson, *Cardiac Auscultation*, Youngstown, Ohio: St. Elizabeth Hospital Medical Center, 1975.)

(carotid pulse) available? Be selective and listen only to S₁. The other sounds can be ignored for now. Practice recording S₁ on an auscultogram.

SELF-LEARNING "UNKNOWN" HEART SOUNDS

On the tape, listen to the "unknown" heart sounds and identify the sound. Compare your answers with the answer key at the end of the chapter. Relisten to the tape as needed to achieve mastery of the content.

1. Is S₁ single or split?

2. Is S₁ single or split?

3. Is S₁ softer or louder than S₂?

4. Is S₁ softer or louder than S₂?

5. Listen to S₁ at the apex, with a bell chest piece and then with a diaphragm chest piece. Is S₁ normal or abnormal?

SELF-LEARNING QUESTIONS

Select the letter of the correct response. Compare your answers with the answer key at the end of the chapter. Reread chapter as needed to achieve mastery of the content.

1. S$_1$ results from
   a. the opening of the mitral valve and tricuspid valve
   b. the closure of the mitral valve and tricuspid valve
   c. the opening of the aortic valve and pulmonic valve
   d. the closure of the aortic valve and pulmonic valve

2. S$_1$'s intensity would be greater or louder if
   a. the chest wall was enlarged
   b. less vigor was behind ventricular contraction
   c. the P-R interval was short
   d. the mitral valve orifice was open and fixed

3. In a normal split S$_1$, how far apart are the closure sounds?
   a. <0.01 second   b. 0.02 to 0.03 second
   c. 0.03 to 0.04 second   d. >0.04 second

4. The normal split S$_1$ is heard best at
   a. base right   b. base left
   c. apex   d. LLSB

5. To differentiate S$_1$ from the S$_2$, which of the following are true?
   (1) At a heart rate of 80 beats per minute or less, S$_1$ follows the longer pause.
   (2) S$_2$ is always loudest at the base.
   (3) With the stethoscope placed on the point of maximal impulse the sound heard simultaneously with the outward thrust is S$_1$.
   (4) The sound heard simultaneously with the palpation of the carotid pulse is S$_1$.
      a. all of the above   b. 1 and 3 only
      c. 3 and 4 only   d. 2 and 4 only

ANSWERS FOR SELF-LEARNING "UNKNOWN" HEART SOUNDS

1. Single S$_1$

2. Split S$_1$

3. Louder S_1

4. Softer S_1

5. Normal S_1 at apex.

ANSWERS FOR SELF-LEARNING QUESTIONS

1. b

2. c

3. b

4. d

5. a

CHAPTER 3
The Second Heart Sound (S₂)

LEARNING OBJECTIVES

After reading this chapter, listening to the accompanying tape, answering the self-learning questions at the end of the chapter, and listening to the "unknowns" on the tape, the learner will be able to do the following:

1. Identify the classical theory for the production of S_2.
2. Differentiate between a single S_2 and a physiological split S_2 (A_2P_2).
3. Identify the physiology behind the normal physiological splitting of S_2.
4. Recognize a normal S_2 at the various auscultatory sites.
5. Differentiate between S_1 and S_2 at the various auscultatory sites.

COMPONENTS OF S₂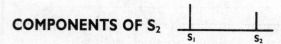

The classical and generally accepted theory for the production of S_2 is due to the closure of both the aortic valve (A_2) and the pulmonic (P_2) valve.

As was true of S_1, the left-sided, mechanical event (A_2) has more energy behind its closure and is therefore louder than the right-sided mechanical event (P_2). Also, the left-sided A_2 normally precedes the right-sided P_2. The A_2 component is discernible at all the auscultatory sites, but is heard best at base right, the site to which aortic sounds radiate best. It is a high-frequency sound, and therefore is heard best with the diaphragm applied firmly.

P_2, the second component making up S_2, is the softer of the two components and is usually only audible at base left, the site to which pulmonic sounds radiate best. It is also a high-frequency sound, and is heard best with the diaphragm applied firmly.

PHYSIOLOGICAL SPLIT S₂

If both components that make up S_2 are separately distinguishable, this is known as a **physiological split**. The normal physiological split of S_2 is heard on inspiration; it becomes single on expiration. Thus respiration normally affects the splitting of S_2 (see Fig. 3-1). In the physiological split S_2, the A_2 and P_2 are about 0.03 second apart. (During inspiration, there is a decrease in intrathoracic pressure that permits an increase in venous return to the right atrium. This increased blood in the right

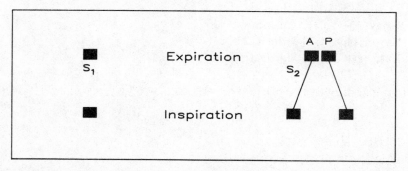

Fig. 3-1. Physiological splitting of the second heart sound (S_2). (Reproduced with permission from L. Caccamo and B. Erickson, *Cardiac Auscultation*, Youngstown, Ohio: St. Elizabeth Hospital Medical Center, 1975.)

atrium prolongs right ventricular systole and delays pulmonic closing. Since P$_2$ occurs further after A$_2$, the split becomes audible.)

Listen now to a physiological split S$_2$—split audible on inspiration; sound single on expiration. A split S$_2$ is normal, or physiological, only if the split occurs during inspiration and becomes single during expiration. It is also normal if the split is not audible. Listen again to an S$_2$ that is split and an S$_2$ that is single (only aortic component audible).

S$_2$ AUSCULTATORY VARIATIONS

Listen now to the normal S$_2$ at the various auscultatory sites:

1. LLSB—single S$_2$
2. Apex—single S$_2$
3. Base right—single S$_2$
4. Base left—split S$_2$ on inspiration; single S$_2$ on expiration

The loudness or intensity of S$_2$ also changes depending on the site auscultated. S$_2$ is always loudest at the base right or base left. It is softer than S$_1$ at the LLSB and the apex.

INTENSITY OF S$_2$

Listen to the loudness of the normal S$_2$ at the various auscultatory sites:

1. LLSB—S$_2$ softer than S$_1$
2. Apex—S$_2$ softer than S$_1$
3. Base right—S$_2$ louder than S$_1$
4. Base left—S$_2$ louder than S$_1$

When listening to the normal S$_2$, the following occurs at each specified site:

1. LLSB—single S$_2$; S$_2$ softer than S$_1$
2. Apex—single S$_2$; S$_2$ softer than S$_1$
3. Base right—single S$_2$; S$_2$ louder than S$_1$
4. Base left—split S$_2$ on inspiration (A$_2$P$_2$); single S$_2$ on expiration (or always single); S$_2$ louder than S$_1$

NORMAL S₁ and S₂

Review now the normal S_1 and S_2 for each specified site:

	S_1	S_2
LLSB	Single or split; louder	Single; softer
Apex	Single; louder	Single; softer
Base right	Single; softer	Single; louder
Base left	Single; softer	Split on inspiration; single on expiration; louder

CLINICAL CORRELATION

When you are confident in your ability to discern S_2, practice it in the clinical area. As you did with S_1, listen to as many different individuals as possible—young, old, thin, fat, etc. Pay special attention to S_2. Can you identify if S_2 is single or physiologically split? Note the difference in intensity depending on the site auscultated. Can you differentiate S_2 from S_1? Listen selectively to S_2, but also listen to S_1. Practice recording both S_1 and S_2 on an auscultogram.

SELF-LEARNING "UNKNOWN" HEART SOUNDS

On the tape, listen to the "unknown" heart souuds and identify the sound. Compare your answers with the answer key at the end of the chapter. Relisten to the tape as needed to achieve mastery of the content.

1. Is S_2 single or physiologically split?

2. Is S_2 single or physiologically split?

3. Is S_1 or S_2 split?

4. Is the S_1 or S_2 split?

5. Listen to S_2 at base right with a bell chest piece and then a diaphragm chest piece. Is S_2 normal or abnormal?

SELF-LEARNING QUESTIONS

Select the letter of the correct response. Compare your answers with the answer key at the end of the chapter. Reread the chapter as needed to achieve mastery of the content.

1. A normal S$_2$ is produced by
   a. the opening of aortic valve and the pulmonic valve
   b. the closing of aortic valve and the pulmonic valve
   c. the opening of the mitral valve and the tricuspid valve
   d. the closing of mitral valve and the tricuspid valve

2. The physiological splitting of S$_2$ relates to the fact that during inspiration
   a. closure of the pulmonic valve is delayed
   b. opening of the pulmonic valve is delayed
   c. closure of the aortic valve is delayed
   d. opening of the aortic valve is delayed

3. In the normal heart, when listening at base right, S$_1$ is single; S$_2$ is
   a. split and softer than S$_1$
   b. split and louder than S$_1$
   c. single and softer than S$_1$
   d. single and louder than S$_1$

4. In the normal heart, when listening at base left, the physiological splitting of S$_2$ will occur during
   a. inspiration
   b. expiration
   c. both inspiration and expiration
   d. neither inspiration nor expiration

5. In the normal heart, S$_2$ is louder than S$_1$ at
   a. LLSB
   b. apex
   c. base right or base left
   d. base left only

ANSWERS FOR SELF-LEARNING "UNKNOWN" HEART SOUNDS

1. Single S$_2$

2. Physiological split S$_2$

3. Split S_1

4. Split S_2

5. Normal S_2 at base right

ANSWERS FOR SELF-LEARNING QUESTIONS

1. b

2. a

3. d

4. a

5. c

CHAPTER 4
The Fourth Heart Sound (S$_4$)

LEARNING OBJECTIVES

After reading this chapter, listening to the accompanying tape, answering the self-learning questions at the end of the chapter, and listening to the "unknowns" on the tape, the learner will be able to do the following:

1. Identify the characteristics of S$_4$.
2. Identify the physiology behind the production of S$_4$.
3. Choose the correct chest piece of the stethoscope for listening to S$_4$.
4. Differentiate right ventricular S$_4$ from left ventricular S$_4$.
5. Differentiate a normal split S$_1$ from an S$_4$.

COMPONENTS OF S₄

S₄ S₁   S₂

S$_4$ is a low-frequency sound heard just before S$_1$. Since it is a sound of **low** frequency it is best heard with the **bell** held lightly. S$_4$ is a result of decreased ventricular compliance or increased volume of filling. It is a sign of ventricular stress.

S$_4$ is a diastolic sound that occurs during the late diastolic filling phase (the time at which "atrial kick" occurs). Ventricles receiving this additional blood from the atrium may generate a low-frequency vibration—the S$_4$. This occurs if the ventricles have a decreased compliance or are receiving an increased diastolic volume. An S$_4$ does not occur unless atrial contraction takes place. Therefore, an S$_4$ is never heard in **atrial fibrillation.**

S$_4$ may be heard normally in a person younger than 20 years of age because of the increased diastolic volume that is normal in the young. S$_4$ also may be indicative of an abnormality of the heart (myocardial infarction is associated with decreased ventricular compliance).

S$_4$ may be of either left ventricular origin or right ventricular origin.

S$_4$ of left ventricular origin is heard best at the apex during expiration, with the patient in the supine or left lateral recumbent position. (Sounds from the left heart radiate best to the apex. Having the patient supine increases the volume of blood in the ventricles making S$_4$ louder. Turning the patient to the left lateral recumbent position brings the heart closer to the chest, also making S$_4$ louder.) Common causes of an S$_4$ of ventricular origin are severe hypertension, aortic stenosis, primary myocardial disease, coronary artery disease, and cardiomyopathy. S$_4$ is heard also in conditions with increased cardiac output and stroke volume such as thyrotoxicosis and anemia. Since S$_4$ is a low-frequency sound, it is heard best with the bell held lightly.

S$_4$ of right ventricular origin is heard best at the LLSB and is accentuated with inspiration. (Sounds from the right heart radiate best to the LLSB. During inspiration, there is an increased volume of blood returned to the right atrium and the right ventricle, making S$_4$ louder.) S$_4$ may reflect pulmonary valve obstruction, pulmonary stenosis, or pulmonic hypertension. Since S$_4$ is a low-frequency sound, it is heard best with the bell held lightly.

Dysrhythmias also may affect the presence or absence of an S$_4$. An S$_4$ may be heard when there is a prolonged P-R interval (0.22 second or longer) and is commonly heard in first, second, or third degree A-V block. It is never heard in atrial fibrillation since atrial contraction does not occur in this dysrhythmia.

An S$_4$ is audible with the bell held lightly. (Pressure on the bell

32

causes the skin to be stretched lightly across the bottom of the bell turning it into a diaphragm.) Thus, firm pressure on the bell will cause an S_4 to diminish or disappear.

Listen now to an S_4. Initially only S_1 and S_2 will be heard; then S_4 will be added. Listen to S_4 with the bell held lightly; then to S_4 with bell applied firmly (note that the S_4 disappears).

DIFFERENTIATING S_4 FROM SPLIT S_1 (M_1T_1)

S_4 has the following characteristics:

1. Low frequency before S_1
2. Heard best with bell held lightly
3. Pressure on bell causes S_4 to diminish or disappear

Split S_1 (M_1T_1) has the following characteristics:

1. High frequency
2. Heard best with diaphragm or bell applied firmly
3. Sounds 0.02 second apart

An S_4 can be decreased by reducing the blood return to the atrium (by standing). An S_4 can be increased by increasing atrial blood return (coughing, squatting, or elevating the legs) or by bringing the heart closer to the stethoscope (by rolling the patient to the left lateral decubitus position).

A split S_1 may be increased on standing but is not significantly affected by other maneuvers.

Again listen to an S_4 compared to a split S_1. Listen to a single S_1; then S_1 split; then an S_4 in front of a split S_1. Then to a split S_1 with an S_4 taken in and out.

CLINICAL CORRELATION

Clinical practice in listening to S_4 can be obtained by selecting patients with conditions most likely to have an S_4. Patients with primary myocardial disease, coronary artery disease, cardiomyopathy, aortic stenosis, or severe hypertension may have an S_4 of left ventricular origin, which is heard best at the apex. An S_4 of right ventricular origin may be heard in a patient with pulmonary valve obstruction, pulmonary stenosis, or pulmonic hypertension. This S_4 is heard best at the LLSB. Coronary care units are an ideal place to hear an S_4 (Remember that patient's with atrial fibrillation cannot have an S_4). Also listen to children who may have an S_4 that is normal. The auscultatory findings between the S_4 in children and the pathological S_4 are similar. The clinical history differentiates the normal S_4 from the pathological S_4.

Don't be discouraged if you have difficulty in hearing an S_4 in the clinical area. S_4 is one of the most difficult sounds to hear since it is just within the ears acoustical ability. To bring out the S_4 have the patient do a mild exercise, such as coughing or turning to the left side. Turning to the left lateral recumbent position also brings the heart closer to the chest wall and makes the S_4 easier to hear. Also listen to S_1 and S_2. Practice recording S_1, S_2, and S_4 on an auscultogram.

SELF-LEARNING "UNKNOWN" HEART SOUNDS

On the tape, listen to the "unknown" heart sounds and identify the sound. Compare your answers with the answer key at the end of the chapter. Relisten to the tape as needed to achieve mastery of the content.

You are listening to the heart at the LLSB:
   Using the bell held lightly, what do you hear?
   Using the bell applied firmly, what do you hear?
   Using the diaphragm, what do you hear?

1. Is S_1 single or split?
   Is there an S_4?

You are listening to the heart at the LLSB:
   Using the bell held lightly, what do you hear?
   Using the bell applied firmly, what do you hear?
   Using the diaphragm, what do you hear?

2. Is S_1 single or split?
   Is there an S_4?

You are listening to the heart at the apex:
   Using the bell held lightly, what do you hear?
   Using the bell applied firmly, what do you hear?
   Using the diaphragm, what do you hear?

3. Is S$_1$ single or split?
   Is there an S$_4$?

   You are listening to the heart at the apex:
   Using the bell held lightly, what do you hear?
   Using the bell applied firmly, what do you hear?
   Using the diaphragm, what do you hear?

4. Is S$_1$ single or split?
   Is there an S$_4$?

   You are listening to the heart at the LLSB:
   Using the bell held lightly, what do you hear?
   Using the bell applied firmly, what do you hear?
   Using the diaphragm, what do you hear?

5. When listening with the bell held lightly:
   Is S$_1$ single or split?
   Is there an S$_4$?

SELF-LEARNING QUESTIONS

Select the letter of the correct response. Compare your answers with the answer key at the end of the chapter. Reread the chapter as needed to achieve mastery of the content.

1. S$_4$ is of
   a. low frequency
   c. medium frequency
   b. high frequency
   d. rough frequency

2. S$_4$ occurs during which phase of the cardiac cycle?
   a. early systolic filling
   c. early diastolic filling
   b. late systolic filling
   d. late diastolic filling

3. You are listening to a patient with atrial fibrillation. You know that an S$_4$ in this patient is
   a. louder than normal
   c. always heard
   b. softer than normal
   d. never heard

4. Which of the following options would you choose to hear an S$_4$ best?
   a. bell applied firmly
   c. diaphragm applied firmly
   b. bell held lightly
   d. diaphragm held lightly

5. An S_4 of left ventricular origin would be heard best at
    a. base right   **b.** base left
    c. apex   **d.** LLSB

ANSWERS FOR SELF-LEARNING "UNKNOWN" HEART SOUNDS

1. Split S_1; no S_4

2. Single S_1; with S_4

3. Single S_1; no S_4

4. Single S_1; with S_4

5. Split S_1; with S_4

ANSWERS FOR SELF-LEARNING QUESTIONS

1. a

2. d

3. d

4. b

5. c

CHAPTER 5
The Third Heart Sound (S₃)

LEARNING OBJECTIVES

After reading this chapter, listening to the accompanying tape, answering the self-learning questions at the end of the chapter, and listening to the "unknowns" on the tape, the learner will be able to do the following:

1. Identify the characteristics of S_3.
2. Identify the physiology behind the production of S_3.
3. Choose the correct chest piece of the stethoscope for listening to S_3.
4. Differentiate a right ventricular S_3 from a left ventricular S_3.
5. Differentiate a physiological split S_2 (A_2P_2) from S_3.
6. Differentiate S_3 from S_4.

COMPONENTS OF S₃

S_3 is a low-frequency sound heard just after S_2. Because it is low frequency, it is heard best with the bell held lightly.

S_3 is a result of decreased ventricular compliance or increased ventricular diastolic volume. It may be a sign of ventricular distress or trouble, as in congestive heart failure. S_3 is a diastolic sound that occurs during the early rapid filling phase of ventricular filling.

S_3 is normal in children and young adults because they have increased diastolic volumes. It is heard in patients with coronary artery disease, cardiomyopathy, incompetent valves, left to right shunts (ventricular septal defects or patent ductus arteriosus and is the **first clinical sign of congestive heart failure.** The above conditions may cause either a decrease in ventricular compliance, an increase in left ventricular diastolic volume, or both.

S_3 may have its origin in either the right or left ventricle—the latter being more common. Left S_3 is heard best at the apex. (Sounds from the left side of the heart are heard best at the apex because this is the area to which they radiate.)

Right S_3 is heard best at the LLSB or xiphoid areas. (Sounds from the right side of the heart are heard best at the LLSB or xiphoid because this is the area to which they radiate.)

Listen now to an S_3. Initially only S_1 and S_2 will be heard; then S_3 will be added.

DIFFERENTIATING S₃ FROM S₄

Timing permits S_3 to be distinguished from S_4:

1. S_3 comes after S_2.
2. S_4 comes before S_1.

In some individuals, both S_3 and S_4 may be present. If the heart rate is normal (60–100 beats per minute), and both S_3 and S_4 are present a **quadruple rhythm** can be heard (four-sound cadence). At a rapid rate, S_3 and S_4 may occur simultaneously and are heard as a very loud diastolic sound known as a **summation gallop.**

For a synopsis of the various sounds that can occur around S_2 and a method of differentiating one from the other, see Table 10–1.

CLINICAL CORRELATION

Clinical practice in listening to S_3 can be obtained by selecting patients with conditions most likely to have an S_3. As was true of S_4, the coronary care unit is one of the best places to hear the pathological S_3. Remember that S_3 is the **first clinical sign of congestive heart failure.** S_3 is normal in children and young adults. The auscultatory findings between the normal S_3 and the pathological S_3 are similar. It is the clinical history that differentiates the two sounds. S_3 is easier to hear than S_4, but you may still need to make S_3 more perceptible by having the patient do a mild exercise, such as coughing or turning to the left side. Changing the patient's position from sitting to supine may also bring out S_3. (This is true of S_4 too.) Also listen to S_1, S_2, and S_4. Can you differentiate the split S_1 from an S_4; the physiological split S_2 from S_3; S_4 from S_3? Practice recording S_1, S_2, S_3, and S_4 on an auscultogram.

SELF-LEARNING "UNKNOWN" HEART SOUNDS

On the tape, listen to the "unknown" heart sounds and identify the sound. Compare your answers with the answer key at the end of the chapter. Relisten to the tape as needed to achieve mastery of the content.

You are listening to the heart at the apex:

Using the bell held lightly, what do you hear?
Using the bell applied firmly, what do you hear?
Using the diaphragm, what do you hear?

1. Is S_2 single, split, or is there an S_3?

You are listening to the heart at base left:
Using the bell held lightly, what do you hear?
Using the bell applied firmly, what do you hear?
Using the diaphragm, what do you hear?

2. Is S_2 single, split, or is there an S_3?

You are listening to the heart at the apex:
Using the bell held lightly, what do you hear?
Using the bell applied firmly, what do you hear?
Using the diaphragm, what do you hear?

3. Is there an S_4 or an S_3?

   You are listening to the heart at the apex:
   Using the bell held lightly, what do you hear?
   Using the bell applied firmly, what do you hear?
   Using the diaphragm, what do you hear?

4. Is there an S_4 or an S_3?

   You are listening to the heart at the apex:
   Using the bell held lightly, what do you hear?
   Using the bell applied firmly, what do you hear?
   Using the diaphragm, what do you hear?

5. Is there an S_4 or an S_3?

SELF-LEARNING QUESTIONS

Select the letter of the correct response. Compare your answers with the answer key at the end of the chapter. Reread the chapter as needed to achieve mastery of the content.

1. S_3 is a low-frequency sound that is heard best with which chest piece of the stethoscope?
   a. bell, held lightly
   b. bell, applied firmly
   c. diaphragm, held lightly
   d. diaphragm, applied firmly

2. S_3 is the result of _____ ventricular compliance or _____ ventricular diastolic volume.
   a. increased; increased
   b. decreased; increased
   c. increased; decreased
   d. decreased; decreased

3. S_3 is heard in an eight-year-old boy with no other abnormal clinical findings. You consider this to be
   a. abnormal, needing consultation
   b. abnormal, watch closely
   c. never normal
   d. normal in children

4. S_3 of left ventricular origin would be best heard at
   a. base right
   b. base left
   c. apex
   d. LLSB

5. The first clinical sign of congestive heart failure is
   a. S_4
   b. wide split S_1
   c. S_3
   d. wide split S_2

ANSWERS FOR SELF-LEARNING "UNKNOWN" HEART SOUNDS

1. Single S_2 with S_3

2. Physiological split S_2

3. S_4

4. S_3

5. S_4 and S_3

ANSWERS FOR SELF-LEARNING QUESTIONS

1. a

2. b

3. d

4. c

5. c

CHAPTER 6
Murmurs—General Information

LEARNING OBJECTIVES

After reading this chapter, listening to the accompanying tape, answering the self-learning questions at the end of the chapter, and listening to the "unknowns" on the tape, the learner will be able to do the following:

1. Define a murmur.
2. Identify the common causes of murmurs.
3. Identify the six characteristics to be considered in murmur identification.
4. Differentiate between murmurs of high, medium, and low frequency.
5. Differentiate between murmurs having the quality of "blow," "harsh," "rough," or "rumble."
6. Differentiate between systolic and diastolic murmurs.

CHARACTERISTICS OF MURMURS

Murmurs are defined as sustained noises that are audible during the time periods of systole, diastole, or both.

Common causes of murmurs include backward regurgitation (a leaking valve, septal defect, or arteriovenous connection); forward flow through a narrowed or deformed valve; a high rate of blood flow through normal or abnormal valves; vibration of loose structures within the heart (chordae tendineae); and continuous flow through A-V shunts.

In order to identify a murmur, there are six characteristics that you need to consider:

1. Location—valve area where murmur is heard best
2. Loudness (intensity)—using the one through six grading system
3. Frequency (pitch)—low, medium, or high
4. Quality—blowing, harsh, rough, or rumble
5. Timing—systolic or diastolic
6. Radiation—where else murmur is heard

Location of Murmurs

The **location of murmurs,** as with normal heart sounds, originates near a heart valve. You will find it necessary to listen to the four basic areas previously discussed plus a fifth area, commonly called Erb's point, which is located at the third intercostal space along the LLSB (see Fig. 6-1).

To determine murmur location, listen to all the basic areas and decide at which area the murmur is heard best. You will find that murmurs from certain valves tend to be heard best "downstream" from the valve as follows:

Valve	Heard Best
1. Mitral	Apex
2. Tricuspid	LLSB
3. Pulmonic	Base left
4. Aortic (systolic)	Base right
Aortic (diastolic)	Erb's point

Loudness of Murmurs

Loudness (intensity) is judged by using the same one through six classification previously discussed for heart sounds.

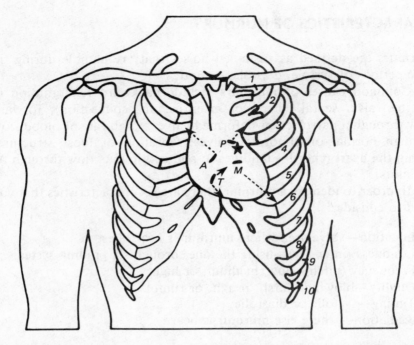

Fig. 6–1. Valve areas: *Anatomic* area is represented by solid bars. M = mitral valve; T = tricuspid valve; A = aortic valve; P = pulmonic valve. *Auscultatory* areas (areas where sound is heard best) are represented by arrows. Star (★) represents Erb's point.

Frequency of Murmurs

Frequency (pitch) indicates whether the sound heard is high, medium, or low. This is easily determined since murmurs of high frequency are heard best with the diaphragm chest piece; those of low frequency with the bell chest piece held lightly; and those of medium frequency with either the bell chest piece or the diaphragm chest piece.

Listen now to murmurs that are considered high, medium, and low.

Quality of Murmurs

Quality is closely related to frequency and is described as "blowing" (mainly high frequency); "harsh" or "rough" (medium frequency—mix of high and low frequencies); and "rumble" (mainly low frequency).

Listen now to murmurs that are described as "blowing," "harsh" or "rough," and "rumble." For a differentiation of the common murmurs by frequency and quality, see Table 6–1.

Table 6–1. Differentiation of common cardiac abnormalities by pitch and quality

Pitch	Frequency (cycles/ sec)	Quality	Abnormality	Chest Piece
High	200–400	Blowing	Mitral regurgitation Tricuspid regurgitation Aortic regurgitation VSD	Diaphragm
Medium	100–200	Harsh	Aortic stenosis	Either
		Rough	Pulmonic regurgitation ASD Increase flow of pulmonary outflow tract	Bell
Low	< 100	Rumble	Mitral stenosis	Bell

Modified with permission from L. Caccamo and B. Erickson, *Cardiac Auscultation,* (Youngstown, Ohio: St. Elizabeth Hospital Medical Center, 1975.)

Timing of Murmurs

Timing means that you can identify whether the sustained noise is occurring between S_1 and S_2—a systolic murmur; or between S_2 and S_1—a diastolic murmur. In some abnormalities, the murmur will be heard both in systole and diastole.

Listen now to a heart rate of 60 beats per minute. First a systolic blow murmur will be added, then removed. Then a diastolic rumble murmur will be added and removed. Murmurs of different frequency and quality have been deliberately selected to help you tell the difference between systole and diastole.

As a beginning auscultator, you may not be able to pinpoint the timing any more precisely than to determine if the murmur occurs in systole or diastole. However, with experience you will note that even **"finer timing"** (early, mid, late, or pan) is possible. A murmur is said to be "early" if its peak intensity occurs early in the cycle; "mid" if the peak intensity occurs in the middle of the cycle; and "late" if the peak intensity occurs late in the cycle. If the murmur is heard throughout the cycle with equal intensity, it is known as a "pan" or "holo" murmur.

Listen now to a heart rate of 60 beats per minute. Then a murmur will be added in the systolic period: early, mid, late, and pan.

Listen now to a heart rate of 60 beats per minute. Then a murmur will be added in the diastolic period: early, mid, late, and pan.

Radiation of Murmurs

Radiation of the murmur is assessed when you determine what other areas the sound is audible besides where you heard it best. Each cardiac abnormality has a classical radiation. See Figures 7–1 and 8–1 for the radiation patterns of common cardiac abnormalities.

SELF-LEARNING "UNKNOWN" HEART SOUNDS

On the tape, listen to the "unknown" heart sounds and identify the sound. Compare your answers with the answer key at the end of the chapter. Relisten to the tape as needed to achieve mastery of the content.

Determine the frequency of the following sustained sounds:

1. This sound is heard best with the diaphragm applied firmly.

2. This sound is heard equally well with either the bell or the diaphragm.

3. This sound is heard best with the bell held lightly.

Determine the quality of the following sounds:

4. This sound is heard best with the diaphragm applied firmly.

5. This sound is heard best with the bell held lightly.

SELF-LEARNING QUESTIONS

Select the letter of the correct response or provide requested information. Compare your answers with the answer key at the end of the chapter. Reread the chapter as needed to achieve mastery of the content.

1. A sustained noise that is audible during the time period of systole, diastole, or both periods is descriptive of a
   a. systolic murmur   b. diastolic murmur
   c. murmur   d. blow

2. Name two common causes for murmur production.
   a.
   b.

3. Name the six characteristics you need to consider in order to identify a murmur.
   a.
   b.
   c.
   d.
   e.
   f.

4. If the sustained noise occurs between S_1 and S_2, the murmur is called
   a. systolic   b. diastolic
   c. regurgitant   d. ejection

ANSWERS FOR SELF-LEARNING "UNKNOWN" HEART SOUNDS

1. High frequency

2. Medium frequency

3. Low frequency

4. Blow

5. Rumble

ANSWERS FOR SELF-LEARNING QUESTIONS

1. c

2. Any two of the following:
   —Backward regurgitation
   —Forward flow thru narrow or deformed valve
   —High rate of blood flow thru normal or abnormal valve
   —Vibration of loose structures within the heart

3. —Location
   —Loudness
   —Frequency
   —Quality
   —Timing
   —Radiation

4. a

CHAPTER 7
Systolic Murmurs

LEARNING OBJECTIVES

After reading this chapter, listening to the accompanying tape, answering the self-learning questions at the end of the chapter, and listening to the "unknowns" on the tape, the learner will be able to do the following:

1. Define a systolic murmur.
2. Identify the mechanism(s) of systolic murmur production.
3. Identify the characteristics of an early, mid-, late, and pan-systolic murmur.
4. Differentiate between an early, mid-, late, and pan-systolic murmur.
5. Identify common adult abnormalities having systolic murmurs.

Systolic murmurs are sustained noises that are audible between S_1 and S_2. In some patients, systolic murmurs may be normal. This may be true of babies or children due to their thin chest walls. In adults a "normal" systolic murmur may be the result of increased blood flow, as in pregnancy.

MECHANISM OF PRODUCTION

Systolic murmurs occur during the ventricular systolic period. Forward flow across the aortic valve or pulmonic valve, or regurgitant flow from the mitral valve or tricuspid valve may produce a systolic murmur. The valves may be normal (but with a high rate of flow) or abnormal. Systolic murmurs may be heard in the normal hearts of children or pregnant women. Common abnormalities having a systolic murmur can include mitral insufficiency, tricuspid insufficiency, aortic stenosis, pulmonic stenosis, and interventricular septal defects.

Early Systolic Murmurs

An **early systolic murmur** begins with S_1 and peaks in the first third of systole. It may be caused by a modified regurgitant murmur with backward flow through an incompetent valve, a septal defect, or an A-V communication. Common causes are a small ventricular septal defect or the innocent murmurs of children.

Listen now to a heart rate of 60 beats per minute. Then an early systolic murmur will be added.

An **innocent systolic** murmur is usually either an **early** murmur or an **ejection** murmur (see midsystolic murmurs). Its grade is a 2/6 or less. It is common in children, and there is no recognizable heart lesion. This sound is considered normal or "innocent" if:

1. Normal split S_2 is heard (S_2 split on inspiration; single on expiration).
2. Normal jugular venous and carotid pulses are present.
3. Normal precordial pulsation is present.
4. Normal history, chest x-ray, and ECG exist.

Common causes are

1. Pulmonary outflow tract murmur (ejection)
2. Vibratory (humming or musical)—heard in children (ages 2 to 7) at the LLSB.

Listen now to a heart rate of 60 beats per minute. Then an early innocent murmur will be added. The early systolic murmur will be compared to a mid-systolic murmur.

Mid-Systolic Murmurs

A **mid-systolic murmur** begins shortly after S_1, peaks in mid-systole, and does not quite extend to S_2. It is known as an "ejection" murmur. It is a crescendo-decrescendo murmur ("diamond-shaped") that builds up and decreases symmetrically. It may be due to forward blood flow through a narrow or irregular valve such as found in aortic stenosis or pulmonic stenosis.

Listen now to a heart rate of 60 beats per minute. Then a midsystolic murmur will be added that is of medium frequency and harsh in quality.

Late Systolic Murmurs

A **late systolic murmur** begins in the latter one half of systole, peaks in the later third of systole, and extends to S_2. It is a modified regurgitant murmur with a backward flow through an incompetent valve. It is heard commonly in papillary muscle disorders and in the mitral valve prolapse syndrome.

Listen now to a heart rate of 60 beats per minute. Then a late systolic murmur will be added that is of high frequency and blowing in quality.

Pan-Systolic (or Holo-Systolic) Murmurs

A **pan-systolic (or holo-systolic) murmur** is heard continuously throughout systole. It begins with S_1 and ends with S_2. Since the pressure remains higher in the ejecting chamber than the receiving chamber throughout systole, the murmur is continuous. It is heard commonly in mitral regurgitation, tricuspid regurgitation, and ventricular septal defect.

Listen now to a heart rate of 60 beats per minute. Then a pan-systolic murmur will be added that is of high frequency and blowing in quality.

For a review of the common adult abnormalities having systolic murmurs see Fig. 7–1.

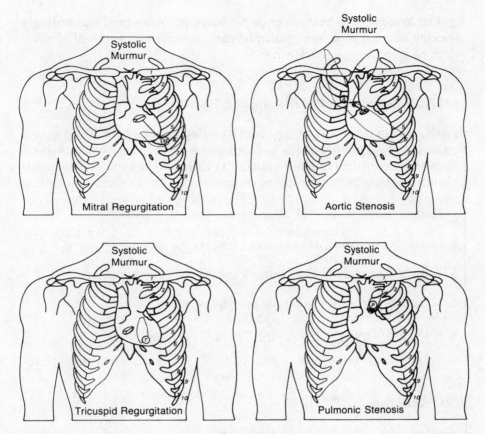

Fig. 7-1. Common cardiac abnormalities with systolic murmur(s): area where murmur is heard best is *circled*; area of usual radiation is *shaded*.

CLINICAL CORRELATION

One of the easiest ways of gaining clinical practice in listening to systolic murmurs is to seek out patients in whom these murmurs already have been identified. Common pathologies with this type of murmur include mitral regurgitation, tricuspid regurgitation, aortic stenosis, and pulmonic stenosis. Patients with mitral valve prolapse may have a late systolic murmur. Systolic murmurs may also be heard in normal hearts, as in the innocent murmur of childhood or pregnancy. Initially try to determine whether the murmur is in systole or diastole. With practice you will be able to tell if it is early, mid, or late in systole. Also determine the following: (1) location—valve area where heard best; (2) loudness; (3) frequency; (4) quality; and (5) radiation. Practice recording the systolic murmur on an auscultogram. Also practice writing a description of the systolic murmur heard.

SELF-LEARNING "UNKNOWN" HEART SOUNDS

On the tape, listen to the "unknown" heart sounds and identify the sound. Compare your answer with the answer key at the end of the chapter. Relisten to the tape as needed to achieve mastery of the content.

Listen to the following systolic murmurs.

1. Is the murmur early, mid-, late, or pan-systolic in nature?

2. Is the murmur early, mid-, late, or pan-systolic in nature?

3. Is the murmur early, mid-, late, or pan-systolic in nature?

4. Is the murmur early, mid-, late or pan-systolic in nature?

5. Is the quality of this late systolic murmur a "blow" or a "rumble"?

SELF-LEARNING QUESTIONS

Select the letter of the correct response. Compare your answers with the answer key at the end of the chapter. Reread the chapter as needed to achieve mastery of the content.

1. Sustained noises that are audible between S_1 and S_2 are descriptive of
   a. systolic murmurs   **b.** diastolic murmurs
   c. ejection sounds   **d.** friction rubs

2. Regurgitant blood flow across which valves will cause a systolic murmur?
   a. mitral and aortic   **b.** mitral and tricuspid
   c. tricuspid and pulmonic   **d.** pulmonic and aortic

3. Forward blood flow across which abnormal valves will cause a systolic murmur?
   a. mitral and aortic   **b.** mitral and tricuspid
   c. tricuspid and pulmonic   **d.** pulmonic and aortic

4. Common adult abnormalities having a systolic murmur include
  a. mitral insufficiency and aortic insufficiency
  b. mitral stenosis and aortic insufficiency
  c. mitral insufficiency and aortic stenosis
  d. mitral stenosis and aortic stenosis

5. A murmur that begins shortly after S_1, peaks in mid-systole, and does not quite extend to S_2 is descriptive of a(n)
  a. early systolic murmur   **b.** mid-systolic murmur
  c. late systolic murmur   **d.** pan-systolic murmur

ANSWERS FOR SELF-LEARNING "UNKNOWN" HEART SOUNDS

1. Early systolic murmur

2. Mid-systolic murmur

3. Pan-systolic murmur

4. Late systolic murmur

5. Blow quality

ANSWERS FOR SELF-LEARNING QUESTIONS

1. a

2. b

3. d

4. c

5. b

CHAPTER 8
Diastolic Murmurs

LEARNING OBJECTIVES

After reading this chapter, listening to the accompanying tape, answering the self-learning questions at the end of the chapter, and listening to the "unknowns" on the tape, the learner will be able to do the following:

1. Define a diastolic murmur.
2. Identify the mechanisms of a diastolic murmur production.
3. Identify the characteristics of an early, mid-, late, and pan-diastolic murmur.
4. Differentiate between an early, mid-, late, and pan-diastolic murmur.
5. Identify common adult abnormalities having diastolic murmur(s).
6. Differentiate between systolic and diastolic murmurs.

Diastolic murmurs are sustained noises that are audible between S_2 and the next S_1. Unlike systolic murmurs, diastolic murmurs usually should be considerd pathological and **not** normal.

MECHANISMS OF PRODUCTION

There are three main **mechanisms of diastolic murmur production:**

1. **Aortic or pulmonic valve incompetence.** During ventricular diastole, the pressure in the ventricles is less than that in the aorta or the pulmonary artery. If the aortic or pulmonic valves are incompetent, then blood regurgitates back into the ventricles. The sustained noise of this regurgitation is the diastolic murmur.
2. **Mitral stenosis or tricuspid stenosis.** During the rapid filling phase of ventricular diastole, if the blood is forced into the ventricles through stenotic valves then a diastolic murmur occurs.
3. **Increased blood flow across mitral valve or tricuspid valve.** If there is an increase in volume or velocity of blood flow across the mitral valve or tricuspid valve during ventricular diastole, a diastolic murmur occurs.

Early Diastolic Murmurs

An **early diastolic murmur** begins with S_2 and peaks in the first third of diastole. It is usually a regurgitant murmur with backward flow through an incompetent valve. Common causes are aortic regurgitation and pulmonic regurgitation.

Listen now to a heart rate of 60 beats per minute. Then an early diastolic murmur will be added that is of high frequency and blowing in quality.

Mid-Diastolic Murmurs

A **mid-diastolic murmur** begins after S_2 and peaks in mid-diastole. Common causes are mitral stenosis and tricuspid stenosis. The murmur is of low frequency and rumbling in quality.

Listen now to a heart rate of 60 beats per minute. Then a mid-diastolic murmur will be added which is of low frequency and rumbling in quality.

Late Diastolic Murmurs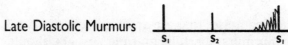

A **late diastolic murmur** begins in the latter one half of diastole, peaks in the later third of systole, and extends to S_1. It is also known as a **presystolic murmur.** It is commonly a component of the murmur of mitral stenosis or tricuspid stenosis. This murmur is of low frequency and rumbling in quality.

Listen now to a heart rate of 60 beats per minute. Then a late diastolic murmur will be added that is of low frequency and rumbling in quality. Listen next to a heart rate of 60 beats per minute. Then a mid-diastolic and a late diastolic murmur will be added that are of low frequency and rumbling in quality.

Pan-Diastolic Murmurs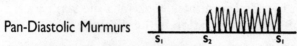

A **pan-diastolic murmur** begins with S_2 and extends throughout the diastolic period. Patent ductus arteriosus, the prototype of aorticopulmonary connections, is a classical example of this murmur. This condition is unusual in an adult, for it is usually corrected in childhood. It usually is heard best at base left and has both a systolic and diastolic component. It is therefore known as a continuous murmur. It may be heard best with the bell chest piece.

Listen next to a heart rate of 60 beats per minute. Then a pan-diastolic murmur will be added that is of low frequency.

Finally, listen to a typical murmur patent ductus arteriosus with both systolic and diastolic components.

For a review of the common adult abnormalities having diastolic murmurs, see Fig. 8–1.

CLINICAL CORRELATION

To gain skill in listening to diastolic murmurs, seek out patients in whom these murmurs have already been identified. Common pathologies having this type of murmur are mitral stenosis, tricuspid stenosis, aortic regurgitation, and pulmonic regurgitation. Initially try to determine whether the murmur is in diastole or systole. Also determine the following: (1) location; (2) loudness; (3) frequency; (4) quality; and (5) radiation. Practice differentiating systolic mumurs from diastolic murmurs. Also practice recording the diastolic murmur on an auscultogram. In addition, write a description of the diastolic murmur heard.

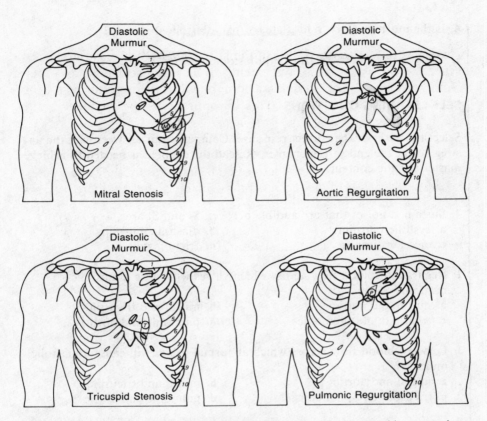

Fig. 8–1. Common cardiac abnormalities with diastolic murmur(s): area where murmur is heard best is *circled*; area of usual radiation is *shaded*.

SELF-LEARNING "UNKNOWN" HEART SOUNDS

On the tape, listen to the "unknown" heart sounds and identify the sound. Compare your answers with the answer key at the end of the chapter. Relisten to the tape as needed to achieve mastery of the content.

Listen to the following diastolic murmurs.

1. Is the murmur early, mid-, late, or pan-diastolic in nature?

2. Is the murmur early, mid-, late, or pan-diastolic in nature?

3. Is the murmur early, mid-, late, or pan-diastolic in nature?

4. Is the murmur early, mid-, late, or pan-diastolic in nature?

5. What is the quality of this mid-diastolic murmur?

SELF-LEARNING QUESTIONS

Select the letter of the correct response. Compare your answers with the answer key at the end of the chapter. Reread the chapter as needed to achieve mastery of the content.

1. Sustained noises that are audible between S_2 and S_1 are
   a. systolic murmurs
   b. diastolic murmurs
   c. ejection sounds
   d. friction rubs

2. Regurgitant blood flow across which valves will cause a diastolic murmur?
   a. mitral and aortic
   b. mitral and tricuspid
   c. tricuspid and pulmonic
   d. pulmonic and aortic

3. Forward blood flow across which abnormal valves will cause a diastolic murmur?
   a. mitral and aortic
   b. mitral and tricuspid
   c. tricuspid and pulmonic
   d. pulmonic and aortic

4. Common adult abnormalities having a diastolic murmur include
   a. mitral stenosis and aortic insufficiency
   b. mitral stenosis and aortic stenosis
   c. mitral insufficiency and aortic insufficiency
   d. mitral insufficiency and aortic stenosis

5. A murmur that begins with S_2 and peaks in the first third of diastole is a(n)
   a. early diastolic murmur
   b. mid-diastolic murmur
   c. late diastolic murmur
   d. pan-diastolic murmur

ANSWERS FOR SELF-LEARNING "UNKNOWN" HEART SOUNDS

1. Mid-diastolic murmur

2. Early diastolic murmur

3. Late diastolic murmur

4. Pan-diastolic murmur

5. "Rumble" quality

ANSWERS FOR SELF-LEARNING QUESTIONS

1. b

2. d

3. b

4. a

5. a

CHAPTER 9
Sounds Around S_1

LEARNING OBJECTIVES

After reading this chapter, listening to the accompanying tape, answering the self-learning questions at the end of the chapter, and listening to the "unknowns" on the tape, the learner will be able to do the following:

1. Differentiate a normal split S_1 (M_1T_1) from a wide split S_1 ($M_1 T_1$).
2. Differentiate a pulmonic ejection sound from an aortic ejection sound.
3. Identify the characteristics of a mid-systolic click.
4. Identify the following:
   a. normal split S_1
   b. wide split S_1
   c. ejection sound—aortic or pulmonic
   d. mid-systolic click
   e. S_4.

WIDE SPLIT S₁

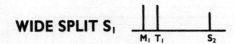

An abnormal split S_1 may result from either electrical or mechanical causes. The resulting asynchrony of the ventricles causes the mitral valve and tricuspid valve closure sounds to be wider apart. The resulting sound is known as a wide split S_1. Electrical causes include conduction problems such as right bundle branch block, ventricular premature beats (especially left), ventricular tachycardia, and third-degree heart block with idioventricular rhythm and, in some, pacing rhythms. Mechanical causes include mitral stenosis, Ebstein's anomaly, and right or left atrial myxomas.

Listen to a wide split S_1 compared with a normal split S_1 and a single S_1.

EJECTION SOUNDS

Ejection sounds are high-frequency "clicking" sounds that occur very shortly after S_1. They usually are heard at either base right or base left. These sounds may be of either *aortic* or *pulmonic* origin and are produced when blood is ejected from the right ventricle or left ventricle either through a stenotic valve or into a dilated chamber. They are heard best with a diaphragm applied firmly because they are high in frequency.

Pulmonic ejection sounds are heard best at base left but may be heard anywhere along the LLSB (see Fig. 9–1A). This sound may increase with expiration and decrease with inspiration in a patient with pulmonary stenosis. The exact reason for this respiratory variation is unknown. It may relate to pressure/volume changes between the right ventricle and pulmonary artery with respiration or be due to the stenosed pulmonary vlave opening with a "snap."

Besides being heard in pulmonic stenosis, the pulmonic ejection sound also may be heard in pulmonary hypertension, atrial septal defects, pulmonary embolism, hyperthyroidism, or in conditions causing enlargement of the pulmonary artery.

Aortic ejection sounds are heard best at the apex but may be heard anywhere on a straight line from base right to the apex. This sound is not affected by respiration. It is heard in valvular aortic stenosis, aortic insufficiency, coarctation of the aorta, and aneurysm of the ascending aorta (see Fig. 9–1B).

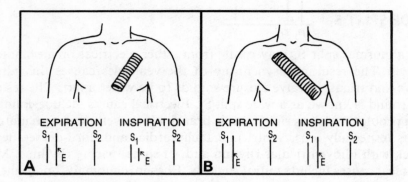

Fig. 9–1. Area for auscultating ejection sounds (E) and respiratory effect: **A**, *pulmonic ejection sound* (E), which decreases in intensity with inspiration and increases in intensity with expiration; **B**, *aortic ejection sound* (E), which is not effected by respiration. (Modified with permission from L. Caccamo and B. Erickson, *Cardiac Auscultation*, Youngstown, Ohio: St. Elizabeth Hospital Medical Center, 1975.)

MID-SYSTOLIC CLICKS

"Clicks" are high-frequency sounds that may be isolated or multiple. While the click usually occurs in the middle of systole, it may also occur in early systole or late systole. It occurs at least 0.14 second after S_1.

The most common cause of a mid-systolic click or clicks is the ballooning of one of the mitral valve leaflets (usually the posterior one) into the left atrium at the point of maximal ventricular ejection. The click is heard when the chordae tendineae, which may be longer than normal, suddenly stop the ballooning leaflet. This is descriptive of mitral valve prolapse and is the most common cause of the mid-systolic click.

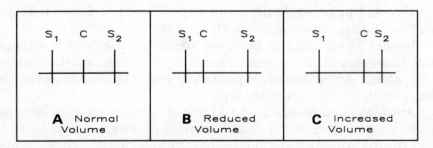

Fig. 9–2. Correlation of click's distance to S_1 and ventricular volume: **A**, *normal* ventricular volume (click in *mid*–systole); **B**, *reduced* ventricular volume (click is *closer* to S_1); **C**, *increased* ventricular volume (click is *farther* from S_1).

Table 9–I. Differential for sounds around the first heart sound (S_1)

Sound Heard	Area Heard Loudest	Respiratory Variation	Chest Piece*	Change c̄ Pressure on Bell	Listen at Base R	
					S_1 Split?	S_2 Split?
Normal Split	LLSB	↑ Inspiration	D	None	No	Normal
RBBB	LLSB	↑ Inspiration	D	None	No	Wide
S_4 Rt	LLSB	↑ Inspiration	B	Decrease	No	Normal
S_4 Lt	Apex	↓ Inspiration ↑ Expiration	B	Decrease	No	Normal
Ejection Pulmonic	Base L	↓ Inspiration ↑ Expiration	D	None	Yes	Wide
Ejection Aortic	Apex	None	D	None	Yes	Wide

*D = diaphragm chest piece; B = bell chest piece.
(Modified with permission from L. Caccamo and B. Erickson, *Cardiac Auscultation*, Youngstown, Ohio: St. Elizabeth Hospital Medical Center, 1975.)

Since the clicks are usually of mitral valve origin, they are heard best at the apex. Or they may be heard toward the LLSB when the posterior leaflet is primarily involved.

Factors that reduce ventricular volume (standing, valsalva, tachycardia, or amyl nitrite) will cause the click to move closer to S_1. (With reduced ventricular volume, the mitral valve closes earlier after S_1 and the click, therefore, moves closer to S_1.)

Factors that increase ventricular volume (squatting, bradycardia, propranolol, pressors) will cause the click to move farther from S_1. With increased ventricular volume, mitral valve closure occurs later and the click, therefore moves further from S_1 (see Fig. 9-2).

For a summary of the various sounds that can occur around S_1 and a method of differentiating one from the other, see Table 9-1.

CLINICAL CORRELATION

In the clinical setting, pay particular attention to S_1 and to "sounds around the first sound." Can you differentiate a normal split S_1 from a wide split S_1; from a mid-systolic click; from ejection sounds—aortic or pulmonic; from S_4? Use Table 9-1 to help you in your differentiation.

SELF-LEARNING "UNKNOWN" HEART SOUNDS

On the tape, listen to the "unknown" heart sounds and identify the sound. Compare your answers with the answer key at the end of the chapter. Relisten to the tape as needed to achieve mastery of the content. You are listening to the heart at base left with the diaphragm, applied firmly:

1. Is S_1 a normal split S_1 or a wide split S_1?

   You are listening to a heart with the diaphragm applied firmly:
   At the LLSB, what do you hear?
   At the apex, what do you hear?
   At base right, what do you hear?
   At base left, what do you hear?

2. The sound you hear around S_1 is a
   a. normal split S_1
   b. wide split S_1
   c. aortic ejection sound
   d. pulmonic ejection sound

You are listening to a heart with the diaphragm applied firmly:
   At the LLSB, what do you hear?
   At the apex, what do you hear?
   At base right, what do you hear?
   At base left, what do you hear?

3. The sound you hear around S_1 is a
   a. normal split S_1 **b.** wide split S_1
   c. aortic ejection sound   **d.** pulmonic ejection sound

You are listening to a heart with the diaphragm applied firmly:
   At the LLSB, what do you hear?
   At the apex, what do you hear?
   At base right, what do you hear?
   At base left, what do you hear?

4. The sound you hear around the S_1 is a
   a. normal split S_1 **b.** wide split S_1
   c. aortic ejection sound   **d.** mid-systolic click

You are listening to the heart at the apex:
   Using the bell held lightly, what do you hear?
   Using the bell applied firmly, what do you hear?
   Using the diaphragm applied firmly, what do you hear?

5. The sound you hear around the S_1 is a
   a. normal split S_1 **b.** aortic ejection sound
   c. S_4 **d.** mid-systolic click

SELF-LEARNING QUESTIONS

Select the letter of the correct response. Compare your answers with the answer key at the end of the chapter. Reread the chapter as needed to achieve mastery of the content.

1. In right bundle branch block or ventricular tachycardia, which of the following will be heard?
   a. normal split S_1 **b.** wide split S_1
   c. pulmonic ejection sound   **d.** mid-systolic click

2. A high-frequency sound that occurs very shortly after S_1 and heard anywhere on a straight line from base right to the apex is descriptive of a
   a. wide split S_1 **b.** mid-systolic click
   c. aortic ejection sound   **d.** pulmonic ejection sound

3. In a mid-systolic click, factors that reduce ventricular volume will cause the click to
   a. disappear   b. become louder
   c. move further from S_1 d. move closer to S_1

4. A wide split S_1 is heard best at
   a. base right   b. base left
   c. apex   d. LLSB

5. A mid-systolic click is heard best at
   a. base right   b. base left
   c. apex   d. LLSB

ANSWERS FOR SELF-LEARNING "UNKNOWN" HEART SOUNDS

1. Wide split S_1

2. c

3. d.

4. d

5. c

ANSWERS FOR SELF-LEARNING QUESTIONS

1. b

2. c

3. d

4. d

5. c

CHAPTER 10
Sounds Around S$_2$

LEARNING OBJECTIVES

After reading this chapter, listening to the accompanying tape, answering the self-learning questions at the end of the chapter, and listening to the "unknowns" on the tape, the learner will be able to do the following:

1. Identify the characteristics of a paradoxical split S$_2$ (P$_2$A$_2$ during expiration).
2. Identify the characteristics of a widely split S$_2$ (A$_2$ P$_2$).
3. Identify the characteristics of a fixed split S$_2$ (A$_2$P$_2$).
4. Identify the characteristics of a narrow split S$_2$ (A$_2$P$_2$).
5. Identify the following:
   a. physiological split S$_2$
   b. paradoxical split S$_2$
   c. wide split S$_2$
   d. fixed split S$_2$
   e. narrow split S$_2$
   f. S$_3$
   g. opening snap.

PARADOXICAL SPLIT S$_2$

$$\text{S}_1 \qquad \text{P}_2\text{A}_2$$

If the closure of the aortic valve is delayed, there may be a reversal of the normal closure sequence of S$_2$ with pulmonic closure (P$_2$) occurring before aortic closure (A$_2$) (see Fig. 10–1).

A paradoxical split S$_2$ is identified clinically when, during inspiration, there is a single S$_2$ and during expiration a split S$_2$. Paradoxical, or reversed, splitting of S$_2$ may occur with marked volume or pressure loads on the left ventricle (severe aortic stenosis, severe aortic regurgitation, and large patent ductus arteriosus). With the increased volume in the left ventricle, ventricular emptying is delayed, thus delaying closure of the aortic valve. It also occurs in conduction defects that delay left ventricular depolarization (complete left bundle branch block). Conduction defects that delay left ventricular depolarization also delay left ventricular emptying, thus also delaying closure of the aortic valve.

Listen now to a paradoxical split S$_2$—split audible on expiration; single on inspiration.

WIDE SPLIT S$_2$

$$\text{S}_1 \qquad \text{A}_2 \text{ P}_2$$

The normal physiological split S$_2$ can be accentuated by conditions that cause an abnormal delay in pulmonic valve closure. Five such conditions are

1. Increased volume in right ventricle as compared with the left (atrial septal defect, ventricular septal defect).

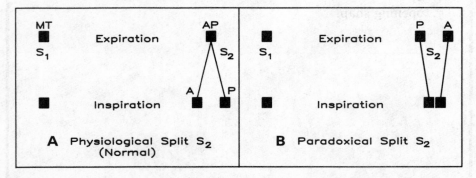

Fig. 10–1. Paradoxical splitting of the second heart sound (S$_2$): **A**, physiological split S$_2$, which splits on *inspiration*, is compared to **B**, paradoxical split S$_2$, which splits on *expiration*. (Reproduced with permission from L. Caccamo and B. Erickson, *Cardiac Auscultation*, Youngstown, Ohio: St. Elizabeth Hospital Medical Center, 1975.)

2. Chronic outflow tract obstruction to the right ventricle (pulmonary stenosis).
3. Acute or chronic dilatation of the right ventricle due to sudden rise in pulmonary artery pressure (pulmonary embolism).
4. Electrical delay or activation of right ventricle (complete right bundle branch block).
5. Decreased elastic recoil of pulmonary artery (idiopathic dilatation of the pulmonary artery).

The wide split has a duration of 0.04 to 0.05 second. The physiological (normal) split is 0.03 second (see Fig. 10–2A).

Listen now to a wide split S_2. Compare it to a normal split S_2 and a single S_2.

FIXED SPLIT S_2

A split that does not change its width with inspiration or expiration is called a fixed split (see Fig. 10–2B). It occurs when the ventricles are unable to change their volumes with respiration. This can occur in congestive heart failure, cardiomyopathy, atrial septal defect, or ventricular septal defect. In congestive heart failure the congested lungs cannot

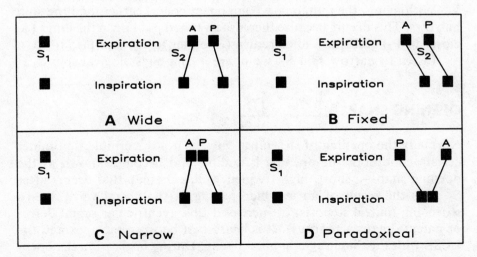

Fig. 10–2. Splitting of the second heart sound (S_2): **A**, wide; **B**, fixed; **C**, narrow; **D**, paradoxical. (Reproduced with permission from L. Caccamo and B. Erickson, *Cardiac Auscultation*, Youngstown, Ohio: St. Elizabeth Hospital Medical Center, 1975.)

withhold much blood from the left ventricle during inspiration, thus left ventricular volume is not affected markedly by respiration. Another factor is that a dilated and poorly compliant left ventricle, which is common to congestive heart failure or cardiomyopathy, may not be able to respond to small changes in volume. Atrial septal defect or ventricular septal defect may prevent the left ventricle alone from changing size on respiration. Or there may be a selective shortening of the left ventricular ejection time with an early aortic closure as in severe mitral insufficiency or ventricular septal defect.

Listen now to a fixed split S_2. Compare it to a physiological split S_2.

NARROW SPLIT S_2

A narrow split S_2 may be heard in conditions that cause increased left ventricular volume without markedly affecting the right side (uncomplicated patent ductus arteriosus with aortic regurgitation). It also may be heard in conditions causing obstruction to outflow of the left ventricle (aortic stenosis or electrical delay as in left bundle branch block). The above conditions would cause delay in the closure of the aortic valve but would not delay closure of the pulmonic valve (A_2 closer to P_2).

With aging, the pulmonary component comes earlier, and the split narrows. This occurs because there is less blood pooling in the lungs (A_2 closer to P_2) and less venous return (P_2 closer to A_2) (see Fig. 10–2C).

Listen to narrow split S_2. Compare it to a physiological split S_2.

OPENING SNAP

Normally the opening of the mitral valve is not discernible, but under certain conditions the opening is audible and becomes known as the opening snap—a short, high-frequency click or snap that occurs after S_2. It is the result of an audible opening of the mitral valve due to stiffening (mitral stenosis) or increased flow (ventricular septal defect or patent ductus arteriosus). It is heard best between the apex and the LLSB with the diaphragm applied firmly. During inspiration the opening snap is softer (because of decreased blood return to left ventricle).

With increased tricuspid flow, as in atrial septal defect, a tricuspid opening snap may be heard. It is a high-frequency sound heard loudest at the LLSB with the diaphragm applied firmly. The tricuspid opening snap becomes louder with inspiration.

DIFFERENTIATING S$_3$ FROM THE OPENING SNAP

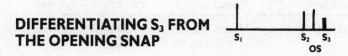

The opening snap occurs earlier after S$_2$ and is a **high** frequency sound best heard with the diaphragm applied firmly. S$_3$ occurs later than the opening snap, following S$_2$, and is a **low**-frequency sound best heard with the bell held lightly.

For a synopsis of the various sounds that can occur around S$_2$ and a method of differentiating one from the other see Table 10–1.

CLINICAL CORRELATION

In the clinical setting, pay particular attention to S$_2$ and the "sounds around the second." Can you differentiate a physiological split S$_2$ from a paradoxical split S$_2$; from a wide split S$_2$; from a fixed split S$_2$; from a narrow split S$_2$; from S$_3$; from an opening snap? Use Table 10–1 to help you in your differentiation.

SELF-LEARNING "UNKNOWN" HEART SOUNDS

On the tape, listen to the "unknown" heart sounds and identify the sound. Compare your answers with the answer key at the end of the chapter. Relisten to the tape as needed to achieve mastery of the content. You are listening to the heart at base left with the diaphragm applied firmly:

1. Is S$_2$ splitting physiologically or paradoxically?

2. Is S$_2$ splitting physiologically or paradoxically?

3. Is S$_2$ wide or narrow?

You are listening to the heart at the apex:
Using the bell held lightly, what do you hear?
Using the bell applied firmly, what do you hear?
Using the diaphragm applied firmly, what do you hear?

Table 10–1. Differential for sounds around the second heart sound (S_2)

Sound Heard	Area Heard Loudest	Respiratory Variation	Chest Piece*	Change c̄ Pressure on Bell
normal split	Base L	Heard on inspiration	D	No
wide split	Base L	Heard on inspiration	D	No
fixed split	Base L	None	D	No
narrow split	Base L	Heard on inspiration	D	No
paradoxical split	Base L	Heard on expiration	D	No
opening snap	Apex or LLSB	↓ inspiration ↑ expiration	D	No
S_3Rt	Xiphoid or LLSB	↑ inspiration	B	Yes
S_3Lt	Apex	↓ inspiration ↑ expiration	B	Yes

*D = diaphragm chest piece; B = bell chest piece.

(Modified with permission from L. Caccamo and B. Erickson, *Cardiac Ausculta-tion,* Youngstown, Ohio: St. Elizabeth Hospital Medical Center, 1975.)

4. Is there an S_3 or a widely split S_2?

You are listening to the heart at the apex:
Using the bell held lightly, what do you hear?
Using the bell applied firmly, what do you hear?
Using the diaphragm applied firmly, what do you hear?

5. Is there an S_3 or an opening snap?

SELF-LEARNING QUESTIONS

Select the letter of the correct response. Compare your answers with the an-swer key at the end of the chapter. Reread the chapter as needed to achieve mastery of the content.

1. The reversal of the normal closure sequence of S_2 with the pulmonic closure (P_2) occurring before aortic closure (A_2) is descriptive of a
   a. physiologically split S_2 **b.** paradoxically split S_2
   c. widely split S_2 **d.** narrowly split S_2

2. Abnormal delay in pulmonic valve closure (P$_2$) is descriptive of a
   a. physiologically split S$_2$ **b.** paradoxically split S$_2$
   c. widely split S$_2$ **d.** narrowly split S$_2$

3. A split S$_2$ that does not change its width with inspiration or expiration is descriptive of a
   a. physiologically split S$_2$ **b.** paradoxically split S$_2$
   c. fixed split S$_2$ **d.** narrowly split S$_2$

4. A split S$_2$ in which the pulmonic component (P$_2$) comes earlier than normal is descriptive of a
   a. physiologically split S$_2$ **b.** paradoxically split S$_2$
   c. fixed split S$_2$ **d.** narrowly split S$_2$

5. A short, high-frequency sound that occurs after S$_2$ and is the result of the audible opening of the mitral valve due to stiffness is descriptive of a
   a. physiologically split S$_2$ **b.** paradoxically split S$_2$
   c. fixed split S$_2$ **d.** opening snap after S$_2$

ANSWERS FOR SELF-LEARNING "UNKNOWN" HEART SOUNDS

1. Physiologically split S$_2$

2. Paradoxically split S$_2$

3. Wide split S$_2$

4. S$_3$

5. Opening snap

ANSWERS FOR SELF-LEARNING QUESTIONS

1. b

2. c

3. c

4. b

5. d

CHAPTER 11
Friction Rubs—Pericardial and Pleural

LEARNING OBJECTIVES

After reading this chapter, listening to the accompanying tape, answering the self-learning questions at the end of the chapter, and listening to the "unknowns" on the tape, the learner will be able to do the following:

1. Identify the common etiologies of a pericardial friction rub.
2. Identify the auscultatory signs of a pericardial friction rub.
3. Identify the sound characteristics of a pericardial friction rub.
4. Identify the common etiologies of a pleural friction rub.
5. Identify the auscultatory signs of a pleural friction rub.
6. Identify the sound characteristics of a pleural friction rub.
7. Differentiate a pericardial friction rub from a pleural friction rub.

To differentiate between pericardial and pleural friction rubs the listener needs to consider the following factors.

PERICARDIAL FRICTION RUBS

Etiologies

A pericardial friction rub is a sign of pericardial inflammation. Some common etiologies include:

1. Infective pericarditis
   Many organisms may cause infective pericarditis.
   Common ones include viral, pyogenic, tubercular, and mycotic.
2. Noninfective pericarditis
   Myocardial infarction, uremia, neoplasms, myxedema, open heart surgery, and trauma are some of the noninfective causes of a pericardial friction rub.
3. Autoimmune problems
   Rheumatic fever, collagen vascular disease, drug induced (i.e., Procainamide) injury, and postmyocardial injury (Dressler's syndrome) are autoimmune causes of pericardial friction.

Auscultatory Signs

The auscultatory signs of a pericardial friction rub are **one systolic sound** and **two diastolic sounds**. The **systolic** sound (between S_1 and S_2) may occur anywhere in systole. The two **diastolic** sounds occur at the times the ventricles are stretched in diastole:

1. In early diastole near the end of the early diastolic filling. (This is the same time when an S_3 would occur.)
2. At the end of diastole, when atrial contraction produces sudden ventricular expansion. (This is the same time that an S_4 would occur.) If atrial contraction does not occur, as in atrial fibrillation, then the second diastolic sound is **not** heard.

Sound Characteristics

1. The pericardial friction rub has a scratching, grating, or squeaking, to-and-fro leathery quality.
2. The pericardial friction rub is *high* in frequency and, therefore, heard best with the *diaphragm* chest piece applied firmly.
3. The pericardial friction rub tends to be louder during **inspiration.** This may be due to the following:
   a. The downward pull of the diaphragm on the pericardium during inspiration, which causes the pericardium to be drawn more tautly over the heart during inspiration.
   b. The expanded lung pressing on the pericardium.
   c. The fact that the pericardium is stretched more during inspiration than during expiration because the expansion of the right ventricle is greater during inspiration than that of the left ventricle during expiration.
4. The pericardial friction rub may be most audible in some patients during **forced expiration** with the patient leaning forward or on hands and knees. (These maneuvers cause less air between the pericardium and the stethoscope and also bring the heart closer to the chest wall.)
5. The pericardial friction rub is likely to be transitory or inconstant. This means that it comes and goes suddenly.
6. The pericardial rub may be heard anywhere on the pericardium but it is often loudest at the LLSB.
7. Most patients with a pericardial friction rub also have tachycardia.

Listen to a pericardial friction rub with a heart rate of 60 beats per minute.

Listen to a heart rate of 60 beats per minute. Then only the systolic component of the rub will be added.

Listen to a heart rate of 60 beats per minute. Then only the diastolic components of the rub will be added.

Now listen to a heart rate of 60 beats per minute. First the systolic component of the rub will be added and then the diastolic components.

Now listen to a pericardial friction rub at a heart rate of 120 beats per minute.

PLEURAL FRICTION RUBS

Etiologies

A pleural friction rub is a sign of pleural inflammation and indicates that the visceral and parietal surfaces of the pleura are rubbing together. Some common etiologies causing pleural friction rubs are

1. Pneumonia
2. Viral infections
3. Tuberculosis
4. Pulmonary embolism

Auscultatory Signs

The auscultatory signs of a pleural friction rub are **one sound during inspiration** and **one sound during expiration** (this may not always be heard).

Sound Characteristics

1. The pleural friction rub has a grating or creaking sound similar to that heard in the pericardial friction rub.
2. The pleural friction rub is *high* in frequency and, therefore, heard best with the *diaphragm* chest piece applied firmly.
3. The pleural friction rub is heard during inspiration and sometimes during expiration. (The expiratory component may be absent.)
4. The pleural friction rub commonly is heard in the lower anterolateral chest wall (the area of greatest thoracic mobility) on the side of the pleural inflammation.
5. The pleural friction rub decreases with a decrease in lung movement. The sound disappears if the breath is held.
6. The pleural friction rub has a superficial character. It sounds closer to the surface than does a pericardial friction rub.

   Listen to a pleural friction rub.
   Listen now to a pleural friction rub with a heart rate of 60 beats per minute.
   Compare the pleural friction rub above to a pericardial friction rub with a heart rate of 60 beats per minute.

Listen again to a pleural friction rub with a heart rate of 60 beats per minute.

Again compare the pleural friction rub above to a pericardial friction rub with a heart rate of 60 beats per minute.

SUMMARY FOR DIFFERENTIATING PERICARDIAL AND PLEURAL FRICTION RUBS

	Pericardial	*Pleural*
Frequency	high	high
Quality	scratching, grating, squeaking	grating or creaking
Chest piece best heard with	diaphragm	diaphragm
Timing	one sytolic sound; two diastolic sounds	one sound inspiration one sound expiration (this may be absent)
	transitory	transitory (but less abrupt)
Site	over pericardium (left chest)	over anterolateral chest—right or left side
Respiratory variant	louder during inspiration	decrease with decrease in breathing; gone when breath held
Surface proximity	further from surface	superficial; closer to surface

CLINICAL CORRELATION

In the clinical setting, seek out patients with pericardial friction rubs and pleural friction rubs. Use the above chart to help you in your differentiation. Compare the sounds of the friction rubs with those of systolic and diastolic murmurs. Practice charting your findings.

SELF-LEARNING "UNKNOWN" HEART SOUNDS

On the tape, listen to the "unknown" heart sounds and identify the sound. Compare your answers with the answer key at the end of the chapter. Relisten to the tape as needed to achieve mastery of the content.

You are listening the LLSB. You hear the following sound.

I. You identify the sound as a

  a. pericardial friction rub   **b.** pleural friction rub
  c. systolic murmur   **d.** diastolic murmur

You are listening to the apex. You hear the following sound.

2. You identify the sound as a

  a. pericardial friction rub   **b.** pleural friction rub
  c. systolic murmur   **d.** diastolic murmur

SELF-LEARNING QUESTIONS

Select the letter of the correct response. Compare your answers with the answer key at the end of the chapter. Reread the chapter as needed to achieve mastery of the content.

I. Identify two of the common etiologies of a pericardial friction rub.
  a.
  b.

2. One of the diastolic sounds of the pericardial friction rub occurs in early diastole; the other occurs at
  a. mid-diastole   **b.** late diastole
  c. rapid diastolic filling   **d.** none of the above

3. Identify two of the common etiologies of a pleural friction rub in early diastole.
  a.
  b.

4. Which characteristic is most helpful in differentiating a pericardial friction rub from a pleural friction rub?
  a. quality   **b.** frequency
  c. breath holding   **d.** site

ANSWERS FOR SELF-LEARNING "UNKNOWN" HEART SOUNDS

I. a

2. b

ANSWERS FOR SELF-LEARNING QUESTIONS

1. Any two of the following:
   —Infective (viral, tuberculosis, etc.)
   —Noninfective (myocardial infarction, etc.)
   —Autoimmune (rheumatic fever, etc.)

2. b

3. Any two of the following:
   —Pneumonia
   —Viral infections
   —Tuberculosis
   —Pulmonary embolism

4. c

REFERENCES

Alspach, JG and Williams, SM: *Core Curriculum for Critical Care Nursing,* ed 3. Philadelphia, W.B. Saunders, 1985.

Caccamo, L and Erickson, B: *Cardiac Auscultation.* Youngstown, Ohio, St. Elizabeth Hospital Medical Center, 1975.

Constant, J: *Bedside Cardiology.* Boston, Little, Brown, 1969.

Erickson, B: Detecting Abnormal Heart Sounds. *Nursing 86,* January, 1986, pp. 58-63.

Harris, A, et al (eds): *Physiological and Clinical Aspects of Cardiac Auscultation.* Philadelphia, J.B. Lippincott, 1976.

Partridge, SA: Cardiac Auscultation. *Dimensions in Critical Care Nursing,* May-June, 1982, pp. 152-156.

Taylor, DL: Assessing Heart Sounds. *Nursing 85,* January, 1985, pp. 51-53.

Visich, M: Knowing What You Hear: A Guide to Assessing Breath and Heart Sounds. *Nursing 81,* November, 1981, pp. 64-76.

GLOSSARY

A₂: Aortic component of the second heart sound. Normally comes before the pulmonic component (P_2).

Aortic ejection sound: See Ejection sound, aortic.

Aortic valve: Semilunar valve that prevents the backflow of blood from the aorta into the left ventricle during ventricular diastole. The closure of this valve is responsible for the first component (A_2) of the second heart sound.

Apex: Area of cardiac auscultation. Also known as the point of maximum impulse (PMI) of the heart against the chest wall. In a normal adult it is at the fifth intercostal space to the left of the sternum at the midclavicular line. Sounds from the mitral valve and the left heart are heard best in this area.

Atrial kick: Slang term for atrial systole or atrial contraction that may contribute 20% to 25% to ventricular filling. It occurs during the late filling phase of the ventricular diastolic period but only if atrial contraction occurs. It can never occur in the presence of atrial fibrillation.

Atrial systole: See Systole, atrial.

Auscultogram: A graphic method of charting heart sounds.

Base left: Area of cardiac auscultation located at the second intercostal space to the left of the sternum. Sounds from the pulmonic valve are heard best in this area.

Base right: Area of cardiac auscultation located at the second intercostal space to the right of the sternum. Sounds from the aortic valve are heard best in this area.

Bell chest piece: A component of the stethoscope that has a shallow shell with a diameter as large as feasible to permit an air seal when held lightly against the chest wall so that no after-imprint is left. It transmits sounds of low frequency.

Cardiac cycle: The period from the beginning of one beat of the heart to the beginning of the next beat. Consists of two phases: one of contraction, systole—atrial and ventricular; and one of relaxation, diastole—atrial and ventricular.

Click: High-frequency sound that is heard after the first heart sound (S_1). It may be a single or multiple sound heard in the middle of the ventricular systolic period. Often associated with mitral valve prolapse.

Compliance: The ratio of change in volume to change in pressure (V/P). Ventricular compliance is decreased in the presence of any condition that limits the ability of the ventricle(s) to expand. Decreased ventricular compliance is one mechanism responsible for the production of the third heart sound (S_3) and the fourth heart sound (S_4).

Diaphragm chest piece: A component of the stethoscope that has a taut (stiff) material drawn across its diameter. When it is applied firmly to the chest wall (leaving an after-imprint), it transmits sounds of high frequency.

Diastole, ventricular: Period of ventricular filling that follows closure of the aortic valve and the pulmonic valve. The ventricular diastolic period is divided into three phases:

1. The first third of the diastolic period has two subdivisions—the isovolumic relaxation phase and the rapid filling phase.
2. The middle third of the diastolic period during which both atrium and ventricles are relaxed.
3. The last third of the diastolic period, or the late filling phase, during which atrial contraction takes place.

Diastolic murmurs: See Murmurs, diastolic.

Duration: The length of time that a sound lasts. Normal heart sounds (S_1 and S_2) are of short duration. Cardiac murmurs or rubs are of long duration.

Ejection murmur: See Murmurs, diastolic, mid.

Ejection sound: A high-frequency "clicking" sound that occurs very shortly after the first heart sound. It may be of either aortic origin or pulmonic origin.

    aortic: High-frequency "clicking" sound heard best at the apex but may be heard anywhere on a straight line from base right to the apex. Heard in valvular aortic stenosis, aortic insufficiency, coarctation of the aorta, and aneurysm of the ascending aorta.

    pulmonic: High frequency "clicking" sound heard best at base left but may be heard anywhere along the left lateral sternal border. Heard in pulmonic stenosis, pulmonary hypertension, atrial septal defect, pulmonary embolism, hyperthyroidism, or in conditions causing enlargement of the pulmonary artery.

First heart sound: The initial sound heard—also known as S_1. It occurs at the beginning of ventricular systole when ventricular volume is maximal. It is due to the closure of the mitral (M_1) valve and the tricuspid (T_1) valve.

    split, normal: When both mitral (M_1) valve closure and tricuspid (T_1) valve closure are distinguishable and 0.02 second apart.

    split, wide: When both mitral valve closure and tricuspid closure sounds occur wider apart from either electrical or mechanical causes which result in ventricular asynchrony.

Fourth heart sound: The fourth heart sound is a low frequency sound heard just before the first heart sound. It is a result of decreased ventricular compliance or increased volume of filling. It is also known as an "atrial gallop," "presystolic gallop," "S_4 gallop," or "S_4."

Frequency: The number of wave cycles generated per second by a vibrating body. It is the vibratory movement of an object in motion that initiates the sound wave cycles that can be discerned by the stethoscope.

  high: The greater the number of wave cycles per second generated by a vibrating body, the higher is the frequency. Sounds of high frequency are best heard with the diaphragm chest piece pressed firmly.

  low: The fewer the number of wave cycles per second generated by a vibrating body, the lower is the frequency. Sounds of low frequency are best heard with the bell applied lightly.

  mid: A combination of high and low frequencies. Sound heard equally well with either bell or diaphragm.

Heart sound simulator: An electronic device designed to generate all normal and abnormal heart sound patterns by the independent variation of all sound parameters.

Intensity: Related to the height of the sound wave produced by a vibrating object. Intensity determines the loudness of the perceived sound. Objects vibrating with great energy are heard as loud sounds. Objects vibrating with low energy are heard as soft sounds.

Isovolumic contraction: A phase during the first part of ventricular systole. It begins with the first initial rise in ventricular pressure after the closure of the mitral valve and the tricuspid valve.

Isovolumic relaxation: A phase during the first third of the ventricular diastole. Initially in this period no blood is entering the ventricles and the ventricles are, therefore, not increasing in volume.

Late filling phase: A phase during the last third of ventricular diastole. The "atrial kick" or atrial contraction takes place at this time.

Left lateral recumbent: Position for cardiac auscultation in which patient is lying on his or her left side with left arm extended under the head, bringing the heart closer to the chest wall. Also the exertion of turning to this position increases heart rate. This position may be useful making the diastolic rumble of mitral stenosis or the low-frequency third heart sound (S_3) of congestive heart failure audible.

Left lateral sternal border (LLSB): Area of cardiac auscultation that is at the fifth intercostal space in the midclavicular line. Sounds from the tricuspid valve and right heart are heard best in this area.

M_1:   The mitral component of the first heart sound. This is normally the first component and occurs just after the mitral valve closes. Normally comes before the tricuspid component (T_1).

Mitral valve: Bicuspid valve between the left atrium and the left ventricle. One of two "A-V valves." Prevents backflow of blood from left ventricle to left atrium during ventricular systole. Closure of this valve is responsible for the first component (M_1) of the first heart sound.

Mitral valve prolapse: Syndrome associated with a midsystolic click and a late systolic murmur. One of the mitral leaflets, usually the posterior one, balloons into the left atrium at the point of maximal ventricular ejection. The click is heard when the chordae tendinae suddenly stop the ballooning leaflet. If the leaflets pull apart, a late systolic murmur of mitral regurgitation may be heard also. Also known as "Barlow's syndrome," "floppy mitral valve," or "click-murmur syndrome."

Murmurs: Sustained noises that are audible during the time periods of systole, diastole, or both:

    diastolic murmur: Sustained noises that are audible between the second heart sound (S_2) and the next first heart sound (S_1). They should be considered organic and not normal. Common causes include mitral stenosis, tricuspid stenosis, aortic regurgitation, and pulmonic regurgitation.

        early: Peaks in the first third of the cycle.

        mid: Peaks in the middle of the cycle. Crescendo-decrescendo ("diamond-shaped"). Also known as "ejection" murmur.

        late: Peaks in the latter third of the cycle.

        pan: Heard continuously throughout the cycle.

    systolic murmur: Sustained noises that are audible between the first heart sound (S_1) and the second heart sound (S_2). Common causes include mitral regurgitation, tricuspid regurgitation, aortic stenosis, and pulmonic stenosis.

Opening snap: A short, high-frequency click or "snap" that occurs after the second heart sound. It is produced most often by the opening of a stenosed, thickened, or distorted mitral valve or tricuspid valve.

P_2:   The pulmonic component of the second heart sound (S_2). Usually follows the aortic component (S_2).

Pitch: A subjective sensation that indicates to the listener whether the tone is high or low on a musical scale.

Point of maximal impulse: Area on the chest where the heart is best palpable. Usually corresponds to the apex, which in a normal adult is located at the fifth intercostal space in the midclavicular line, to the left of the sternum.

Pulmonic ejection sound: See ejection sound, pulmonic.

Pulmonic valve: Semilunar valve that prevents backflow of blood from the pulmonary artery into the right ventricle during ventricular diastole. Closure of the valve is responsible for the second component (P_2) of the second heart sound.

Quality: This is a sound characteristic that distinguishes two sounds with equal degrees of frequency and intensity but which come from a different source (piano from a violin or heart from lung).

    blow: Mainly high-frequency.

    harsh: Mix of high and low frequencies—slightly more high than low.

    rough: Mix of high and low frequencies—slightly more low than high.

    rumble: Mainly low-frequency.

Rapid filling phase: A phase during the first third of ventricular diastole. It occurs when ventricular pressure is less than atrial pressure. The mitral valve and tricuspid valve then open and blood rapidly enters the ventricles.

Rapid ventricular ejection: A phase during the first part of ventricular systole. It follows the isovolumic contraction phase. It occurs when ventricular pressure exceeds the pressure in the aorta and the pulmonary artery, and forces the aortic valve and pulmonic valve open causing blood to be rapidly ejected from the ventricles.

S_1:   See first heart sound.

S_2:   See second heart sound.

S_3:   See third heart sound.

S_4:   See fourth heart sound.

Second heart sound: The second sound heard in a normal heart—also known as S_2. It occurs at the end of ventricular systole. It is due to the closure of the aortic (A_2) valve and the pulmonic (P_2) valve.

    split, fixed: This split does not change its width with inspiration or expiration.

    split, narrow: The aortic (A_2) component and the pulmonic (P_2) component are closer together than normal—< 0.03 second. The split is heard on inspiration and is single on expiration.

    split, paradoxical: Reversal of the normal closure sequence of the second heart sound (S_2) with pulmonic closure (P_2) occurring before aortic closure (A_2). This split is heard during expiration and becomes single on inspiration. (The opposite of a normal or physiological split.)

    split, physiological: The aortic (A_2) component and pulmonic (P_2) component that make up the second sound are distinguishable separately—0.03 second apart. The split is heard on inspiration and becomes single on expiration.

    split, wide: Delay in pulmonic valve closure can cause the physiological split to be accentuated or increased—0.04 to 0.05 second. The split is heard during inspiration and becomes single on expiration.

Sine wave: An up and down, or to and fro undulating or wavy line.

Split: When both components that make up a sound are separately distinguishable, the sound is said to "split." A duration of 0.02 second between the sounds is necessary in order for the ear to be able to make this distinction. See also First heart sound, split and Second heart sound, split.

Stethoscope: Acoustical instrument that utilizes the vibration of sounds reacting upon the air column enclosed in tubing to transmit sounds to the listener's ear. When used for heart sounds a bell chest piece and diaphragm chest piece are necessary.

Systole, atrial: Period in cardiac cycle. It occurs during the last third of ventricular diastole or during the late filling phase. During this period contraction of the atrium takes place and the remaining blood is squeezed from the atrium. This is also known as the "atrial kick." Atrial systole may contribute 20% to 25% to ventricular filling. The contribution is less at faster heart rates—100 beats per minute or greater.

Systole, ventricular: Period in cardiac cycle that follows closure of the mitral valve and tricuspid valve. This systolic period is divided into two phases. The first phase includes the isovolumic contraction phase and the rapid ventricular ejection phase. During the latter part of ventricular systole, ventricular pressure falls and reduced ventricular ejection occurs. This second phase lasts until ventricular ejection stops and ventricular diastole begins.

Systolic murmurs: See Murmurs, systolic.

T_1: The second component of the first heart sound. It normally occurs after M_1 (the mitral component) just after the tricuspid valve closes.

Third heart sound: A low-frequency sound heard just after the second heart sound. It is a diastolic sound that occurs during the early rapid filling phase of ventricular diastole. It is a result of decreased ventricular compliance or increased ventricular diastolic volume. It is also known as a "ventricular gallop," "protodiastolic gallop," "S_3 gallop," or an "S_3."

Thrill: A continuous palpable sensation felt on the precordium. It is comparable to the vibration felt when a cat purrs.

Thrust: A palpable (sometimes even visible) intermittent sensation. This is the sensation felt when palpating the point of maximal impulse (PMI) at the apex of the heart.

Timing: Determining whether a sound is occurring during the systolic period or the diastolic period.

   finer: Determinig whether a sound is occurring early, mid-, or late in the systolic period or diastolic period.

Tricuspid valve: The three-leaflet valve between the right atrium and the right ventricle. One of two "A-V" valves. Prevents backflow of blood from the right ventricle to right atrium during ventricular systole. Closure of this valve is responsible for the second component (T_1) of the first heart sound.

Turbulence: Smooth blood flow is disturbed and the blood flows crosswise in the vessel or chamber as well as along the vessel. This causes eddy currents, similar to a whirlpool, and produces vibrations that are audible.

Ventricular diastole: See Diastole, ventricular.

Ventricular systole: See Systole, ventricular.

INDEX